Acknowledgements

I am very grateful to the following colleagues for providing me with illustrations:

Prof. A. Bird (Figs 52, 220, 221, 246, 248, 252); R. Marsh (Fig. 64); T. Rahman (Figs 138, 203); J. Shilling (Fig. 134); A. Shun-Shin (Figs 46, 50, 127, 235, 249); D. Taylor (Fig. 169); V. Tanner (Fig. 45); B. Mathalone (Figs 72, 254, 262, 263); J. Federman (Fig. 232); D. Spalton (Fig. 130); P. Morse (Fig. 238); C. Migdal (Figs 68, 69, 240).

10 0316850 2

COLOUR

Ophthalmology

Jack J. Kanski MD MS FRCS FRCOphth
Consultant Ophthalmic Surgeon
Prince Charles Eye Unit
King Edward VII Hospital
Windsor

SECOND EDITION

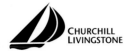

CHURCHILL
LIVINGSTONE

EDINBURGH LONDON NEW YORK PHILADELPHIA SYDNEY
TORONTO 1997

University of Nottingham
at Derby Library

CHURCHILL LIVINGSTONE
An imprint of Harcourt Publishers Limited

🏝 is a registered trademark of Harcourt Publishers Limited

Text:
© Longman Group Ltd 1984, 1992
This edition © Pearson Professional Limited 1997
© Harcourt Brace and Company Limited 1998
© Harcourt Publishers Limited 2001
Illustrations:
© Jack J. Kanski 1984, 1992, 1997
J. J. Kanski has asserted his right under the
Copyright, Designs and Patents Act, 1998, to be
identified as Author of this work.

All rights reserved. No part of this publication
may be reproduced, stored in a retrieval system,
or transmitted in any form or by any means,
electronic, mechanical, photocopying, recording
or otherwise, without either the prior permission
of the publishers (Harcourt Publishers Limited,
Robert Stevenson House, 1-3 Baxter's Place, Leith
Walk, Edinburgh EH1 3AF), or a licence permitting
restricted copying in the United Kingdom issued
by the Copyright Licensing Agency, 90 Tottenham
Court Road, London, W1P 0LP, UK.

First published as Colour Aids Ophthalmology
1984
First Colour Guide edition 1992
Second Colour Guide edition 1997
  Reprinted 1998
  Reprinted 2001

ISBN 0 443 05804 0

British Library Cataloguing in Publication Data
A catalogue record for this book is available from
the British Library.

**Library of Congress Cataloging in Publication
Data**
A catalog record for this book is available from
the Library of Congress.

Medical knowledge is constantly
changing. As new information
becomes available, changes in
treatment, procedures, equipment
and the use of drugs become
necessary. The author and the
publishers have, as far as it is
possible, taken care to ensure
that the information given in this
text is accurate and up to date.
However, readers are strongly
advised to confirm that the
information, especially with
regard to drug usage, complies
with current legislation and
standards of practice.

The
publisher's
policy is to use
**paper manufactured
from sustainable forests**

Printed in China

For Churchill Livingstone

Publisher: Michael Parkinson
Project editor: James Dale
Project controller: Nancy Arnott
Design direction: Erik Bigland

Contents

1 / Chronic blepharitis

Clinical features

Staphylococcal anterior blepharitis
This is a very common infection of the base of the lashes which causes chronic ocular irritation. It is very common in patients with atopic eczema (Fig. 1).

Signs: anterior lid margins are red and scaly (Fig. 2). The scales are brittle and are centred around the base of the lashes. In long-standing cases there is loss of lashes (madarosis) and the remaining ones become misdirected (Fig. 3).

Common associated findings: mild papillary conjunctivitis (see Fig. 62), punctate epitheliopathy, tear film instability, recurrent styes (see Fig. 10) and marginal keratitis (see Fig. 104).

Seborrhoeic anterior blepharitis
This is a disorder of the glands of Zeis and typically affects patients with seborrhoeic dermatitis. It may occur in isolation or in association with either staph. blepharitis or posterior blepharitis.

Signs: anterior lid margins are red and waxy. The scales are soft and greasy and, in contrast to staph. blepharitis, are found in between the lashes. The lashes are frequently stuck together (Fig. 4).

Posterior blepharitis
This is caused by dysfunction of meibomian glands and is common in patients with acne rosacea or seborrhoeic dermatitis.

Signs: posterior lid margins are red and distorted (Fig. 5). The meibomian gland orifices may be capped by oil (Fig. 6). Expressed meibomian secretions may be turbid or semi-solid (like toothpaste), and the tear film may be frothy. The meibomian gland ductules within the tarsal plate may be distorted and scarred. Recurrent meibomian cyst formation (see Fig. 7) is common.

Management

- *Lid hygiene* with diluted (25%) baby shampoo to remove crusts and scales.
- *Topical treatment* with antibiotic ointment.

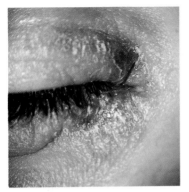

Fig. 1 Eczema of the eyelids.

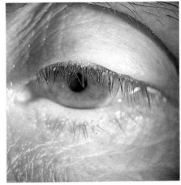

Fig. 2 Scales at base of eyelashes.

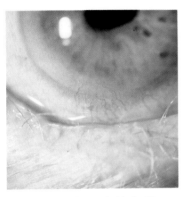

Fig. 3 Long-standing staph. blepharitis.

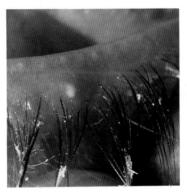

Fig. 4 Inflammation of eyelid margin and sticking together of eyelashes.

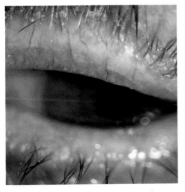

Fig. 5 Combined anterior and posterior blepharitis of upper lid.

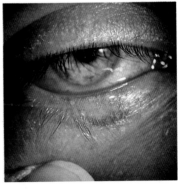

Fig. 6 Oily globules at meibomian gland orifices.

Meibomian cyst (chalazion)

This common condition is caused by meibomian gland dysfunction with secondary lipogranulomatous inflammation. It occurs with increased frequency in patients with seborrhoeic dermatitis and acne rosacea. It presents with a chronic, painless, non-tender, roundish, firm swelling in the tarsal plate (Fig. 7) which may be associated with a secondary conjunctival granuloma (Fig. 8).

Treatment: surgical incision and curettage is usually required.

Internal hordeolum (acute chalazion)

This is a purulent infection of a meibomian gland. It presents with an acutely painful and tender, inflamed swelling within the tarsal plate (Fig. 9). Severe cases may be associated with mild preseptal cellulitis.

Treatment: incision and curettage may be required after the acute infection has resolved.

External hordeolum (stye)

This is a small abscess of a gland of Zeis or Moll which presents as a tender inflamed localized swelling on the lid margin which points through the skin (Fig. 10).

Treatment: removal of the associated eyelash and hot spoon bathing to promote discharge.

Cyst of Zeis

This is a chronic, painless, small, opaque, smooth, cystic nodule on the lid margin (Fig. 11). A cyst of Moll is similar but translucent.

Molluscum contagiosum

These are single or multiple, small, pale, waxy umbilicated nodules (Fig. 12) which may be associated with an ipsilateral chronic follicular conjunctivitis (see Fig. 57).

1003168502

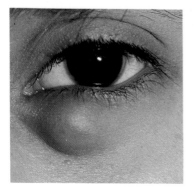

Fig. 7 Large meibomian cyst.

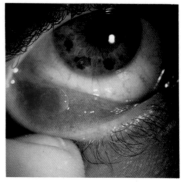

Fig. 8 Conjunctival granuloma secondary to meibomian cyst.

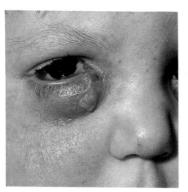

Fig. 9 Internal hordeolum.

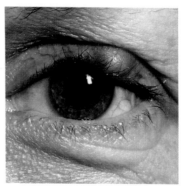

Fig. 10 External hordeolum (stye).

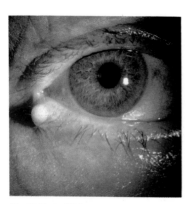

Fig. 11 Cyst of Zeis.

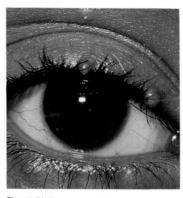

Fig. 12 Molluscum contagiosum.

3 / Benign tumours of the eyelids

Clinical types

Squamous cell papilloma
This is the most common benign tumour of the eyelid. It has a characteristic raspberry-like surface and it may be broad based (sessile) or pedunculated (Fig. 13). The tumour should be differentiated from actinic keratosis and squamous cell carcinoma which may also have a papillary configuration.

Basal cell papilloma (seborrhoeic keratosis)
This common tumour is usually found in the elderly. It is a discrete, greasy, brownish lesion with a friable verrucous surface which appears to be stuck to the skin (Fig. 14).

Keratoacanthoma
This presents as a fast-growing, firm, pinkish nodule which develops rolled edges and a keratin-filled crater (Fig. 15). It remains stationary for a few months and, unless removed, it spontaneously involutes.

Acquired naevi
- *Junctional naevus*—flat, well circumscribed lesion with a uniform brown colour.
- *Compound naevus*—elevated lesion with a homogenous tan to brown colour.
- *Dermal naevus*—elevated lesion with variable pigmentation (Fig. 16).

Capillary haemangioma (strawberry naevus)
This typically develops in infancy as an irregular slightly raised red lesion which, if large, may cause a mechanical ptosis (Fig. 17). It may also involve the orbit (see Fig. 43). Unless treated, it frequently involutes by the age of 3 years.

Plexiform neurofibroma
This rare tumour typically occurs in patients with neurofibromatosis type-1 and may be associated with ispilateral glaucoma. It characteristically gives rise to a mechanical ptosis and an S-shaped deformity (Fig. 18).

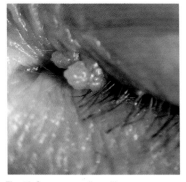

Fig. 13 Squamous cell papilloma.

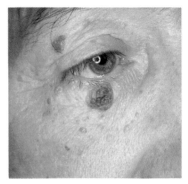

Fig. 14 Seborrhoeic keratosis.

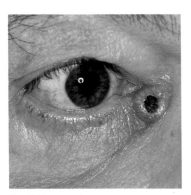

Fig. 15 Keratocanthoma.

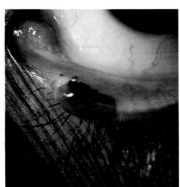

Fig. 16 Dermal naevus.

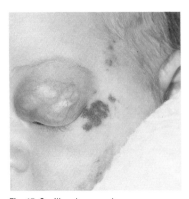

Fig. 17 Capillary haemangioma.

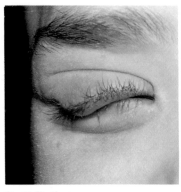

Fig. 18 Plexiform neuroma.

Clinical types

Basal cell carcinoma

Basal cell carcinoma (BCC) is the most common eyelid malignancy. It is locally invasive but does not metastasize. 50% of BCCs involve the lower lid and 30% the medial canthus. The main clinical types are:

- *Nodular BCC* is an indurated nodule with fine surface blood vessels (Fig. 19)—associated hyperkeratosis may give the tumour a pearly appearance
- *Noduloulcerative BCC (rodent ulcer)* has raised, rolled edges and central ulceration (Fig. 20)
- *Sclerosing BCC* is a flat indurated plaque with poorly demarcated margins and loss of overlying lashes (Fig. 21).

Squamous cell carcinoma

Squamous cell carcinoma (SCC) is much less common than BCC. It grows faster and may metastasize. The tumour may arise de novo or from a premalignant dermatosis such as actinic keratosis, Bowen's disease and xeroderma pigmentosum. The main clinical types are:

- *Nodular SCC* starts as a hyperkeratotic nodule or plaque and then develops crusting fissures
- *Ulcerating SCC* resembles a rodent ulcer (Fig. 22)
- *Papillary SCC* may resemble a benign papilloma.

Sebaceous gland carcinoma

This is a rare but very aggressive tumour. The main clinical types are:

- *Meibomian gland carcinoma*: a diffuse, hard swelling within the tarsal plate (Fig. 23) that may be mistaken for a meibomian cyst
- *Gland of Zeis carcinoma*: a discrete, firm, yellowish nodule on the lid margin (Fig. 24)
- *Spreading sebaceous gland carcinoma*: infiltrates the dermis and may also spread within the conjunctival epithelium (Pagetoid spread) and may mimic 'chronic conjunctivitis' or 'superior limbic keratoconjunctivitis' (see Fig. 39).

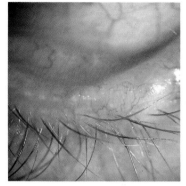

Fig. 19 Nodular basal cell carcinoma.

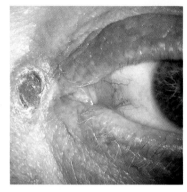

Fig. 20 Rodent ulcer.

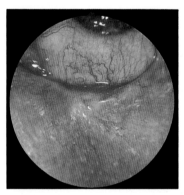

Fig. 21 Sclerosing basal cell carcinoma.

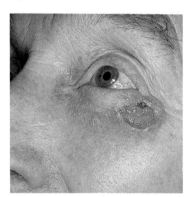

Fig. 22 Squamous cell carcinoma.

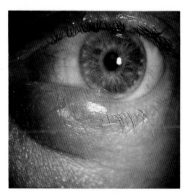

Fig. 23 Meibomian gland carcinoma.

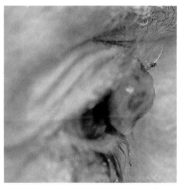

Fig. 24 Gland of Zeis carcinoma.

5 / Ptosis

Neurogenic ptosis

- *Third nerve palsy* causing paralysis of the levator (Fig. 25).
- *Horner syndrome*: mild ptosis associated with miosis (Fig. 26). Anhydrosis is present if the lesion is below the superior cervical ganglion and heterochromia may occur if the lesion is congenital.
- *Misdirection of third nerve*: bizarre movements of the upper lid which accompany various eye movements. Typically follows an acquired 'surgical' third nerve palsy.
- *Marcus Gunn jaw-winking syndrome*: congenital, uncommon, ptosis associated with retraction of the lid induced by stimulation of ipsilateral pterygoids.

Aponeurotic ptosis

- *Involutional*: age-related laxity of the levator aponeurosis (Fig. 27).
- *Postoperative*: stretching of the aponeurosis during surgery.

Mechanical ptosis

- *Excessive weight*: oedema, tumours (see Figs 17 & 18) or redundant skin.
- *Cicatricial*: reduced mobility from severe scarring of the upper lid skin or conjunctiva.

Myogenic ptosis

- *Simple congenital*: bilateral or unilateral (Fig. 28). The ptotic lid is higher than the normal in downgaze due to poor relaxation. There may also be superior rectus weakness.
- *Blepharophimosis syndrome*: rare, bilateral congenital ptosis, associated with telecanthus, epicanthus inversus and lower lid ectropion (Fig. 29).
- *Acquired*: myasthenia gravis, ocular myopathy or myotonic dystrophy (Fig. 30).

Treatment

If possible the cause should be treated (e.g. myasthenia gravis). Surgical options, depend on the type and severity of ptosis.

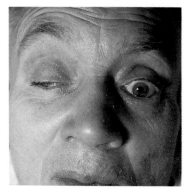

Fig. 25 Severe ptosis due to third nerve palsy.

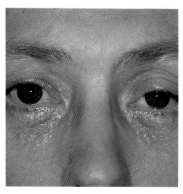

Fig. 26 Mild left ptosis in Horner syndrome.

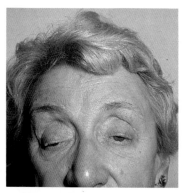

Fig. 27 Severe bilateral involutional ptosis.

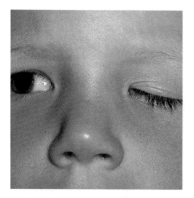

Fig. 28 Severe left congenital ptosis.

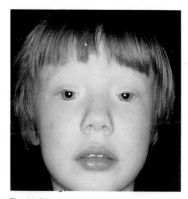

Fig. 29 Blepharophimosis syndrome.

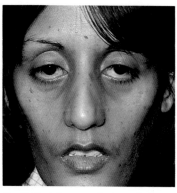

Fig. 30 Ptosis in myotonic dystrophy.

Clinical features

Entropion

This is an inversion of the eyelid.

- *Involutional entropion* is very common and is caused by age-related changes (Fig. 31). It involves only the lower lid and, if severe and prolonged, may result in corneal scarring and vascularization (Fig. 32).
- *Cicatricial entropion* (Fig. 33) is caused by scarring of the palpebral conjunctiva which may occur in chronic trachoma or ocular pemphigoid (see Fig. 76).
- *Acute spastic entropion* only involves the lower lid and is frequently temporary. It is caused by spasm of the orbicularis muscle as a result of ocular irritation or essential blepharospasm.
- *Congenital entropion* is very rare and only involves the lower lid.

Ectropion

This is an outward turning of the eyelid which mostly involves the lower lid. If severe and prolonged, it may cause conjunctival keratinization (Fig. 34).

- *Involutional ectropion* is caused by age-related changes.
- *Cicatricial ectropion* is caused by scarring of skin and underlying tissues resulting from burns or following resection of tumours (Fig. 35).
- *Mechanical ectropion* is caused by large lower lid tumours.
- *Paralytic ectropion* is caused by a facial nerve palsy. It is associated with incomplete blinking and inability to completely close the lids.
- *Congenital ectropion* is caused by shortage of skin. It may be associated with the blepharophimosis syndrome (see Fig. 29).

Trichiasis

This is an inward misdirection of lashes which, if severe, may cause corneal irritation and scarring (Fig. 36).

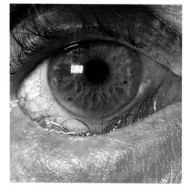

Fig. 31 Involutional entropion.

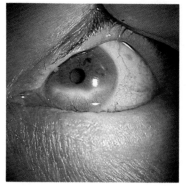

Fig. 32 Entropion of lower eyelid with corneal vascularization and scarring.

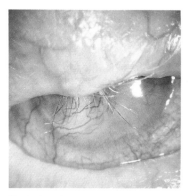

Fig. 33 Cicatricial entropion.

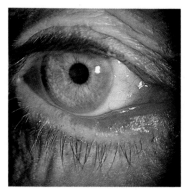

Fig. 34 Ectropion of the lower eyelid with conjunctival keratinization.

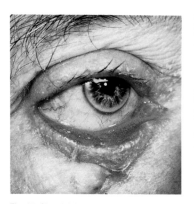

Fig. 35 Cicatricial ectropion.

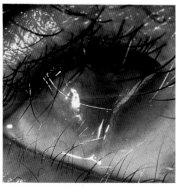

Fig. 36 Trichiasis in trachoma.

Clinical features

Eyelid signs
- Lid retraction in primary position—Dalrymple's sign (Fig. 37).
- Lid lag in downgaze—von Graefe's sign.
- Staring and frightened appearance—Kocher's sign.

Soft tissue involvement
- Fullness of the eyelids.
- Conjunctival injection and chemosis (Fig. 38).
- Superior limbic keratoconjunctivitis characterized by superior tarsal papillary hypertrophy, hyperemia of the superior bulbar conjunctiva, (Fig. 39), and superior corneal filaments.

Proptosis
This is typically axial and may be unilateral, bilateral, or asymmetrical (Fig. 40). Severe proptosis may prevent adequate lid closure and give rise to exposure keratopathy. Fundus examination may show choroidal folds (Fig. 41).

Restrictive myopathy
In order of frequency, the four motility defects are
- defective elevation (tight inferior rectus—Fig. 42)
- defective abduction (tight medial rectus)
- defective depression (tight superior rectus)
- defective adduction (tight lateral rectus)

Optic neuropathy
This very serious complication is caused by compression of the optic nerve or its blood supply by enlarged extraocular muscles.

Symptoms: slowly progressive impairment of visual acuity associated with defective red–green appreciation.

Signs
- Afferent pupillary conduction defect.
- Disc edema, although in some cases the disc may be normal.
- Visual field defects.

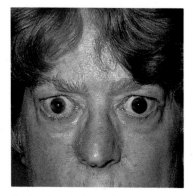

Fig. 37 Bilateral lid retraction.

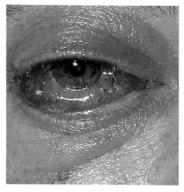

Fig. 38 Severe chemosis due to thyroid ophthalmopathy.

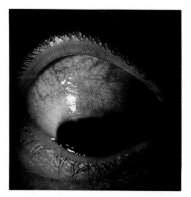

Fig. 39 Superior limbic keratoconjunctivitis.

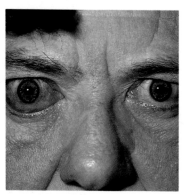

Fig. 40 Right proptosis.

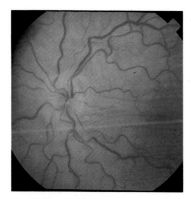

Fig. 41 Choroidal folds.

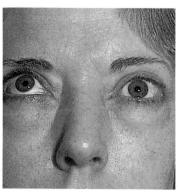

Fig. 42 Defective elevation of the left eye.

14

8 / Orbital tumors

Clinical types

Hemangiomas

- *Capillary hemangioma:* presents in infancy with an anterior orbital swelling (Fig. 43) that increases in size when infant is crying. A "strawberry nevus" on the eyelids (see Fig. 17) may be an associated finding. The tumor enlarges and then usually spontaneously diminishes in size.
- *Cavernous hemangioma:* most common benign orbital tumor in adults. It presents in young adults with a gradual onset of painless axial proptosis, which may be associated with choroidal folds (see Fig. 41).

Orbital varices

Presentation
- Intermittent nonpulsatile proptosis.
- Visible lesions (Fig. 44).
- Combination of visible lesions and proptosis.
- Acute orbital hemorrhage or thrombosis.

Rhabdomyosarcoma

This malignant tumor presents at about the age of 7 years with a subacute onset of painful progressive proptosis. Examination typically shows a superonasal mass, although any part of the orbit may be involved (Fig. 45).

Neural tumors

- *Optic nerve glioma* presents in childhood with slowly progressive proptosis and visual loss. The optic disc may be swollen or pale (see Fig. 241). Between 25–50% of patients have associated neurofibromatosis type 1.
- *Optic nerve sheath meningioma* causes slowly progressive visual loss followed later by proptosis (Fig. 46). The optic disc frequently shows opticociliary shunt vessels (Fig. 47).

Dermoid cysts

- *Superficial dermoids* present in infancy with a firm, round mass in the anterior orbit (Fig. 48).
- *Deep dermoids* present in adolescence or adult life with nonaxial proptosis.

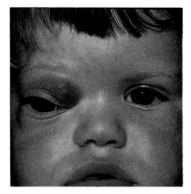

Fig. 43 Capillary hemangioma.

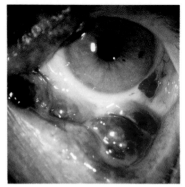

Fig. 44 Orbital varices.

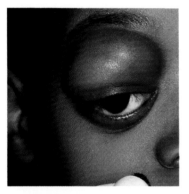

Fig. 45 Rhabdomyosarcoma.

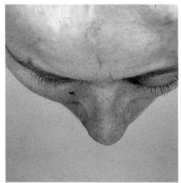

Fig. 46 Left proptosis due to meningioma.

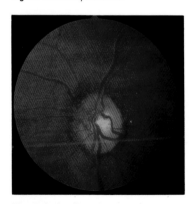

Fig. 47 Opticociliary shunt vessels.

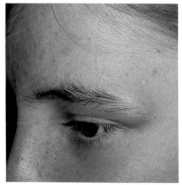

Fig. 48 Orbital dermoid cyst.

Clinical types

Orbital cellulitis

This is the result of infection of the soft tissues of the orbit behind the orbital septum. The main types are

- *Sinus-related:* usually secondary to childhood ethmoidal sinusitis
- *From adjacent structures:* e.g., dacryocystitis
- *Post-traumatic*
- *Postsurgical:* retinal, orbital, or lacrimal surgery

Signs: acute onset of lid edema (Fig. 49), chemosis, proptosis, painful ophthalmoplegia, and pyrexia.

Orbital pseudotumor

This is a rare idiopathic inflammation that may affect any of the soft tissues of the orbit.

Signs: subacute onset of usually unilateral pain, lid edema, chemosis, proptosis (Fig. 50), and ophthalmoplegia.

Carotid-cavernous fistula

Causes
- *Fracture* of the base of the skull.
- *Spontaneous rupture* of an internal carotid artery into the cavernous sinus.

Signs: sudden onset chemosis (Fig. 51), dilated conjunctival vessels (Fig. 52), pulsatile proptosis, ophthalmoplegia, raised intraocular pressure (IOP), and dilated retinal veins and hemorrhages (Fig. 53).

Blow-out fracture of orbital floor

This is caused by a blow to the orbit by an object greater in diameter than 5 cm.

Signs: periorbital edema and ecchymosis, enophthalmos (Fig. 54), vertical diplopia, and infraorbital nerve anesthesia.

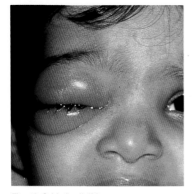

Fig. 49 Orbital cellulitis.

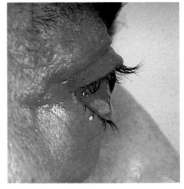

Fig. 50 Orbital pseudotumor.

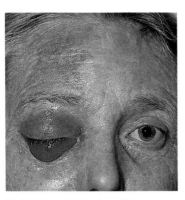

Fig. 51 Chemosis in patient with a spontaneous carotid-cavernous fistula.

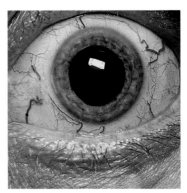

Fig. 52 Dilated blood vessels due to carotid-cavernous fistula.

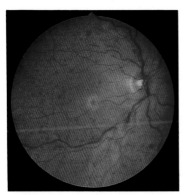

Fig. 53 Dilated retinal vein and hemorrhages in carotid-cavernous fistula.

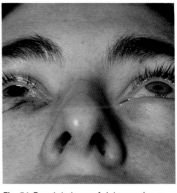

Fig. 54 Enophthalmos of right eye due to severe blow-out fracture of orbital floor.

Clinical features

Seasonal allergic (hay fever) conjunctivitis

This is characterized by an acute onset of bilateral itching, lid edema, and chemosis (Fig. 55).

Bacterial conjunctivitis
This very common and self-limiting condition presents with a subacute onset of bilateral but frequently asymmetrical redness, grittiness, and discharge. The eyelids are frequently stuck together on waking.

Signs: conjunctival infection that is most intense in the fornices, and variable discharge (Fig. 56).

Adenoviral conjunctivitis
This common infection is very contagious and can be spread by finger-to-eye contact or by contaminated ophthalmic instruments.

Signs: acute onset of frequently bilateral discomfort and a watery discharge associated with follicular conjunctivitis (Fig. 57) and preauricular lymphadenopathy. In severe cases, there may be lid edema, chemosis, subconjunctival hemorrhages (Fig. 58), and pseudomembranes. In some cases, a punctate epithelial keratitis develops. The corneal lesions may either resolve spontaneously or progress to deeper infiltrates (Fig. 59).

Neonatal conjunctivitis
This is defined as a conjunctival inflammation that occurs within the first month of life.

Causes
- *Chlamydial conjunctivitis* presents between days 5–14 and is the most common (Fig. 60).
- *Gonococcal conjunctivitis* presents between days 1–3.
- *Herpes simplex conjunctivitis* presents between days 5–7.
- *Simple bacterial conjunctivitis* presents at any time.

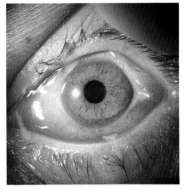

Fig. 55 Hay fever conjunctivitis.

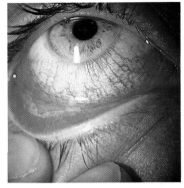

Fig. 56 Bacterial conjunctivitis.

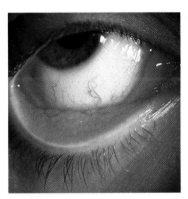

Fig. 57 Follicular conjunctivitis due to adenoviral infection.

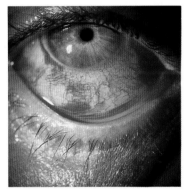

Fig. 58 Subconjunctival hemorrhage in severe adenoviral infection.

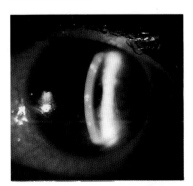

Fig. 59 Anterior stromal corneal infiltrates.

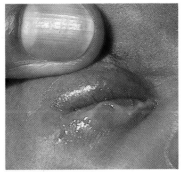

Fig. 60 Mucopurulent discharge in newborn due to chlamydial infection.

Clinical types

Adult inclusion conjunctivitis
This is caused by a venereal chlamydial infection.

Signs: usually unilateral mucopurulent discharge associated with large conjunctival follicles, preauricular lymphadenopathy, and subepithelial infiltrates. A corneal micropannus may develop in severe cases (Fig. 61).

Vernal keratoconjunctivitis (spring catarrh)
This is a bilateral chronic recurrent disease that starts in childhood. It is common in patients with other features of atopy (i.e., asthma, eczema, and hay fever).

Signs: chronic itching, lacrimation, photophobia, and a stringy discharge associated with a papillary conjunctivitis mainly involving the superior tarsus (Fig. 62). Nodules at the limbus (limbitis) occur in some cases (Fig. 63).

Complications: punctate epitheliopathy, macroerosions, plaque formation (Fig. 64), subepithelial scarring, persistent epithelial defects, and occasionally a "cupid bow" limbal scarring (pseudogerontoxon—Fig. 65).

Atopic keratoconjunctivitis
This rare but potentially serious condition typically affects young men with atopic dermatitis.

Signs: eyelids are thickened, crusted, and fissured (see Fig. 1). The conjunctiva shows infiltration and papillary hypertrophy (see Fig. 62).

Complications: symblepharon (see Fig. 77), punctate epitheliopathy, epithelial defects, shield-shaped stromal scars, and peripheral neovascularization.

Giant papillary conjunctivitis
This is a foreign body–associated conjunctivitis characterized by giant papillae on the superior tarsus (Fig. 66). It may be caused by contact lenses, artificial eyes, and protruding sutures.

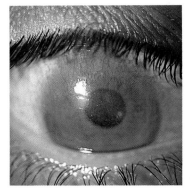

Fig. 61 Superior micropannus.

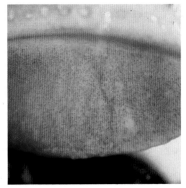

Fig. 62 Papillary conjunctivitis.

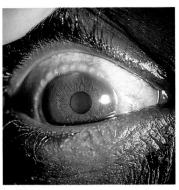

Fig. 63 Vernal limbitis.

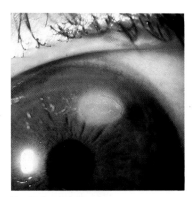

Fig. 64 Corneal plaque.

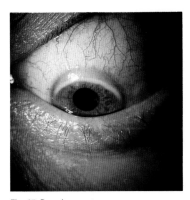

Fig. 65 Pseudogerontoxon.

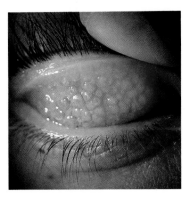

Fig. 66 Giant papillae.

Pigmented tumors

Conjunctival nevus
This presents during childhood or early adult life as a single, well-demarcated, flat or slightly elevated lesion with variable pigmentation. The limbus is the most common site (Fig. 67).

Primary acquired melanosis
This very rare condition presents during late life with unilateral, unifocal or multifocal slowly growing patches of intraepithelial pigmentation.

Melanoma
- *Primary melanoma* presents as a solitary pigmented or nonpigmented raised nodule most frequently located at the limbus (Fig. 68).
- *Arising from primary acquired melanosis*, which is characterized by the development of nodular lesions within areas of pre-existing melanosis (Fig. 69).

Nonpigmented tumors

Papilloma
- *Pedunculated papilloma* typically affects children and young adults and may be unilateral or bilateral.
- *Sessile papilloma* affects older patients and is invariably single and unilateral (Fig. 70).

Carcinoma
- *Intraepithelial carcinoma* is characterized by slightly elevated, fleshy vascular, or a gelatinous avascular mobile mass (Fig. 71).
- *Invasive carcinoma* has a similar appearance but is fixed to underlying tissues.

Choristoma
- *Dermoid* is a solid white mass most frequently located at the limbus (Fig. 72).
- *Lipodermoid* is a soft yellow movable subconjunctival mass.

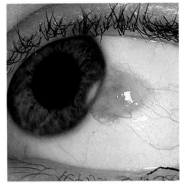

Fig. 67 Conjunctival nevus.

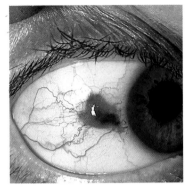

Fig. 68 Primary conjunctival melanoma.

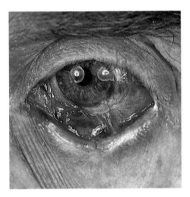

Fig. 69 Melanoma arising from primary acquired melanosis.

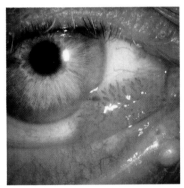

Fig. 70 Sessile conjunctival papilloma.

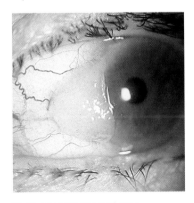

Fig. 71 Intraepithelial carcinoma.

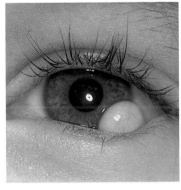

Fig. 72 Limbal dermoid.

Classification

Keratoconjunctivitis sicca (KCS)

This is caused by atrophy of lacrimal tissue.

- *Idiopathic KCS*, in which the lacrimal glands alone are affected.
- *Sicca complex*—associated with a dry mouth (xerostomia).
- *Primary Sjögren syndrome*—xerostomia and serologic evidence of an autoimmune process.
- *Secondary Sjögren syndrome*—associated with a connective tissue disorder.

Signs: thin marginal tear strip filled with mucous debris, corneal filaments, and mucus (Fig. 73). Rose bengal stains the dry conjunctiva and cornea (Fig. 74). Tear film break-up time is reduced, and Schirmer's test shows decreased wetting.

Cicatrizing conjunctivitis

This very serious but rare condition may be associated with one of the following:

- *Cicatricial pemphigoid* is characterized by blisters of skin and mucous membranes.
- *Stevens–Johnson syndrome* is an acute, severe, but generally self-limiting vesiculobullous disease. The oral mucosal lesions characteristically cause hemorrhagic crusting of the lips (Fig. 75). Ocular complications are usually less severe than in cicatricial pemphigoid.

Signs: advanced disease: conjunctival scarring (Fig. 76) and shrinkage, adhesions between the bulbar and palpebral conjunctiva (symblepharon—Fig. 77), adhesions at the outer canthi (ankyloblepharon), dry eye, metaplastic lashes, and cicatricial entropion (see Fig. 33). Severe corneal damage is secondary to keratinization, ulceration, infection, and vascularization (Fig. 78).

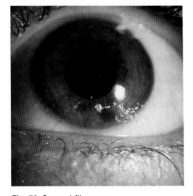

Fig. 73 Corneal filaments.

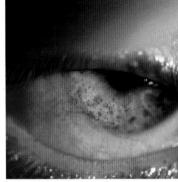

Fig. 74 Staining with rose bengal.

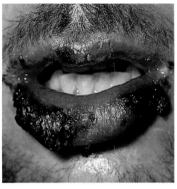

Fig. 75 Hemorrhagic crusting of lips in Stevens–Johnson syndrome.

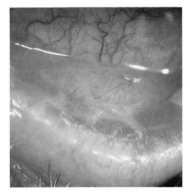

Fig. 76 Conjunctival scarring in cicatricial pemphigoid.

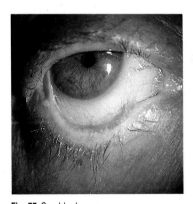

Fig. 77 Symblepharon.

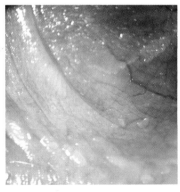

Fig. 78 Corneal changes in cicatricial pemphigoid.

Clinical types

Bacterial keratitis

This is usually associated with pre-existing corneal surface disease or contact lens wear.

Signs: circumcorneal injection, stromal infiltration, and an overlying epithelial defect. A hypopyon may be present if secondary anterior uveitis is severe. The configuration of the stromal infiltration to a certain extent depends on the causative organism as follows:

- *Staph and pneumococcal keratitis:* oval, yellow-white, suppuration surrounded by relatively clear cornea (Figs. 79 and 80).
- *Pseudomonas keratitis:* irregular suppuration associated with a mucopurulent discharge (Figs. 81 and 82).

Fungal keratitis

Signs: the clinical appearance to a certain extent depends on the infectious agent.

- *Filamentous keratitis* is frequently preceded by ocular trauma with vegetable matter. It is characterized by grayish white ulceration with indistinct feathery margins surrounded by finger-like satellite lesions (Fig. 83).
- *Candida keratitis* typically occurs in debilitated patients or eyes with pre-existing surface disease. The appearance is similar to bacterial keratitis.

Acanthamoeba keratitis

This typically occurs in contact lens wearers.

Signs: blurred vision and pain that is characteristically disproportionate to the clinical signs. Early cases are characterized by dendritiform epithelial lesions, radial keratoneuritis, and stromal keratitis. In established cases, there is a non-suppurative ring associated with variable epithelial breakdown (Fig. 84).

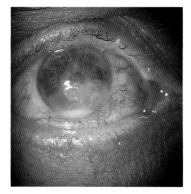

Fig. 79 Staph keratitis.

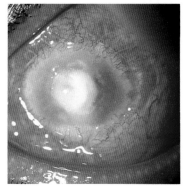

Fig. 80 Advanced pneumococcal keratitis with hypopyon.

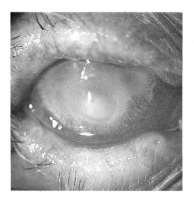

Fig. 81 Advanced pseudomonas keratitis.

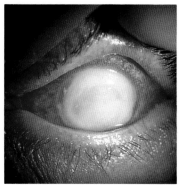

Fig. 82 Complete corneal opacification in pseudomonas keratitis.

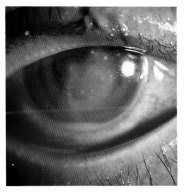

Fig. 83 Fungal keratitis with hypopyon.

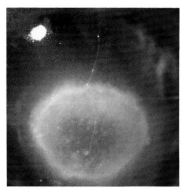

Fig. 84 *Acanthamoeba* keratitis.

Clinical types

Primary infection

This is caused by direct transmission of virus through infected secretions to a nonimmune subject. It may cause follicular conjunctivitis (see Fig. 57), blepharitis (Fig. 85), and epithelial keratitis.

Recurrent epithelial keratitis

This common condition is caused by invasion of the epithelium by reactivated latent virus.

Signs
- *Dendritic ulcer* starts with coarse stellate punctate epithelial lesions that develop into a branching ulcer. Fluorescein stains the bed of the ulcer (Fig. 86) and rose bengal its margins. Corneal sensation is diminished.
- *Geographic (amoeboid) ulcer* starts as a dendritic ulcer and enlarges (Fig. 87).

Treatment: with topical antiviral agents.

Stromal necrotic keratitis

This uncommon condition is caused by direct viral invasion and destruction of the stroma.

Signs: cheesy necrotic stroma similar to bacterial or fungal infection (Fig. 88). Complications include vascularization and scarring (Fig. 89).

Treatment: aimed at healing any associated epithelial defect and then diminishing stromal inflammation by the judicious use of topical steroids with antiviral and antibiotic cover.

Disciform keratitis

This common condition is caused by a hypersensitivity reaction to the virus. It presents with subacute, painless blurring of vision, which may be associated with seeing halos around lights.

Signs: a central area of epithelial edema and stromal thickening (Fig. 90). Associated findings include folds in Descemet's membrane, mild iritis with small keratic precipitates, and a ring of infiltrates surrounding the lesion (Wessley ring).

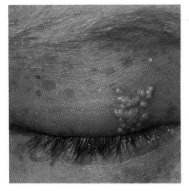

Fig. 85 Primary herpes simplex lesions.

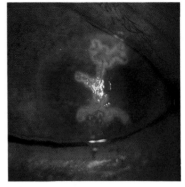

Fig. 86 Large dendritic ulcer stained.

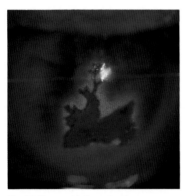

Fig. 87 Geographic herpetic ulcer.

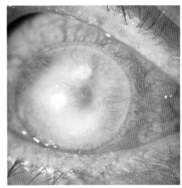

Fig. 88 Stromal necrotic keratitis.

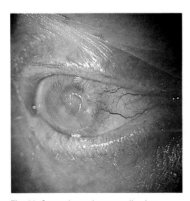

Fig. 89 Corneal scarring complicating stromal keratitis.

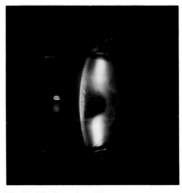

Fig. 90 Disciform keratitis.

Herpes zoster (shingles) is caused by the zoster-varicella virus. Approximately 15% of all cases of herpes zoster affect the ophthalmic division of the trigeminal nerve (herpes zoster ophthalmicus). Ocular involvement is common when the rash involves the side of the nose (Hutchinson's sign).

Clinical features

Skin lesions

The initial rash is maculopapular and then becomes vesicular. The vesicles subsequently burst to form crusting ulcers. The skin lesions are usually associated with variable periorbital edema (Fig. 91).

Treatment
- *Systemic therapy* with oral antiviral agents curtails vesiculation, accelerates healing, and reduces neuralgia, but only if administered early.
- *Topical therapy* with antiviral creams and paints as well as steroid-antibiotic preparations should be used until the crusts have separated.

Ocular complications
- *Conjunctivitis and episcleritis* are the most common acute lesions which resolve spontaneously within 1 week.
- *Acute keratitis* may be of the following types: punctate epithelial, filamentary (see Fig. 73), microdendritic, nummular (Fig. 92), and disciform (see Fig. 90).
- *Chronic corneal lesions* include mucus plaque keratitis, secondary lipid keratopathy (Fig. 93) and neurotropic keratitis, which may lead to perforation (Fig. 94).
- *Acute iritis* is common. It may give rise to secondary elevation of IOP and segmental iris atrophy (Fig. 95).
- *Scleritis* (Fig. 96) is uncommon and frequently also involves the cornea (sclerokeratitis).
- *Neuro-ophthalmologic complications* include optic neuritis and extraocular nerve palsies.

Treatment: iritis and most acute corneal lesions are treated with topical steroids.

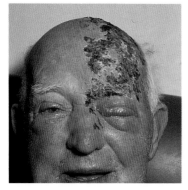

Fig. 91 Severe herpes zoster ophthalmicus.

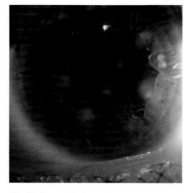

Fig. 92 Nummular keratitis.

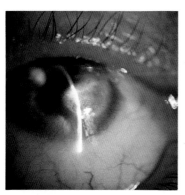

Fig. 93 Lipid keratopathy.

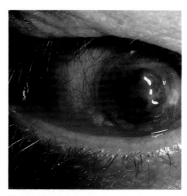

Fig. 94 Very severe corneal thinning.

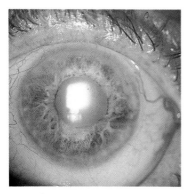

Fig. 95 Segmental iris atrophy after herpes zoster iritis.

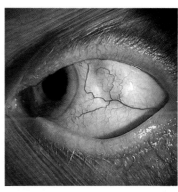

Fig. 96 Scleral thinning due to past herpes zoster scleritis.

17 / Corneal dystrophies

Clinical features

Cogan's microcystic dystrophy
Presentation of this common and relatively innocuous dystrophy is during the third decade of life, with symptoms of recurrent corneal erosions characterized by acute pain, lacrimation, and photophobia on waking.

Signs: bilateral, subtle, dot-like, cystic (Fig. 97) or linear-like epithelial lesions that do not affect visual acuity.

Reis–Bücklers' dystrophy
Presentation of this dominantly inherited dystrophy is during the first decade of life, with recurrent corneal erosions.

Signs: bilateral, ring-like opacities at the level of Bowman's layer, which give the cornea a "honeycomb" appearance (Fig. 98).

Lattice dystrophy
Presentation of this dominantly inherited dystrophy is during the first decade of life, with recurrent corneal erosions.

Signs: delicate network of overlapping spider-like deposits involving the anterior and mid stroma (Fig. 99).

Granular dystrophy
Presentation of this dominantly inherited dystrophy is during the first or second decades of life, either with recurrent erosions or mild visual impairment.

Signs: very small, discrete, crumb-like granules within the anterior stroma (Fig. 100).

Fuchs' endothelial dystrophy
Presentation is between the fifth and seventh decades of life with visual impairment.

Signs: bullous keratopathy associated with stromal edema (Fig. 101). Severe cases may require corneal grafting (Fig. 102).

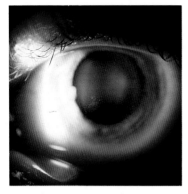

Fig. 97 Corneal erosions in Cogan's microcystic dystrophy.

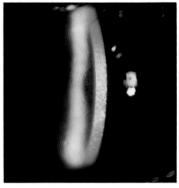

Fig. 98 Reis–Bücklers' dystrophy.

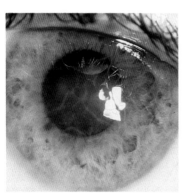

Fig. 99 Lattice dystrophy.

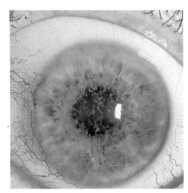

Fig. 100 Granular dystrophy.

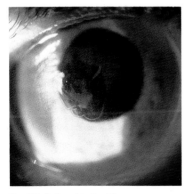

Fig. 101 Bullous keratopathy.

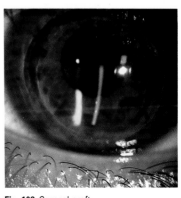

Fig. 102 Corneal graft.

Clinical types

Dellen

Signs: saucer-like thinning secondary to local stromal dehydration most frequently associated with elevated limbal lesions (Fig. 103).

Treatment: if possible, the cause should be eliminated and rehydration promoted by patching and lubricants.

Marginal keratitis
This very common condition is caused by a hypersensitivity to staphylococcal exotoxins. It may be associated with chronic staph blepharitis (see Fig. 2).

Signs: subepithelial infiltrate separated from the limbus by clear cornea (Fig. 104). It may spread circumferentially and be associated with subsequent epithelial breakdown.

Rosacea keratitis
This occurs in about 5% of patients with acne rosacea.

Signs: inferior punctate epitheliopathy followed by peripheral vascularization (Fig. 105) associated with subepithelial infiltration. Severe peripheral thinning and perforation may occur but are uncommon.

Severe peripheral ulceration

Causes
- Mooren's ulcer is an idiopathic, very rare, but serious condition that may be unilateral or bilateral. When advanced, the ulceration may involve the entire circumference of the cornea and may also spread centrally (Fig. 106).
- Associated with rheumatoid arthritis—ulceration may be chronic and not associated with inflammation (contact lens cornea—Fig. 107) or it may be acute and associated with severe inflammation at the limbus (Fig. 108).

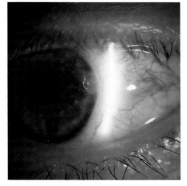

Fig. 103 Corneal dellen.

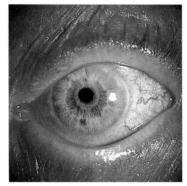

Fig. 104 Marginal keratitis.

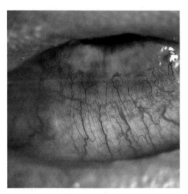

Fig. 105 Rosacea keratitis.

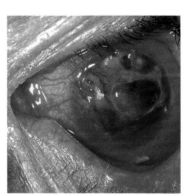

Fig. 106 Advanced Mooren's ulcer.

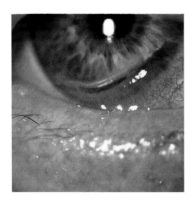

Fig. 107 Corneal thinning in rheumatoid arthritis.

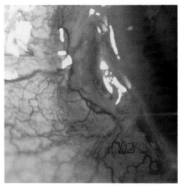

Fig. 108 Corneal ulceration in rheumatoid arthritis.

Clinical types

Keratoconus

This is a common cone-like bulging of the central cornea (Fig. 109). It presents during the second or third decades of life, with slowly progressive blurring of vision from irregular astigmatism. Both eyes are affected in 85% of cases.

Signs
- *Early:* abnormal fundoscopy reflex, irregular "scissors" retinoscopy reflex, and fine vertical lines in the deep stroma (Vogt's striae—Fig. 110).
- *Late:* iron deposits at the base of the cone (Fleischer's ring), bulging of the lower lid in downgaze (Munson's sign), central corneal edema (acute hydrops—Fig. 111), and corneal scarring.

Systemic associations: atopic dermatitis, osteogenesis imperfecta, and syndromes: Down, Turner, Ehlers–Danlos, and Marfan.

Treatment: initially with contact lenses. Advanced cases require corneal grafting (see Fig. 102).

Keratoglobus

Very rare congenital bilateral thinning and protrusion of the entire cornea (Fig. 112).

Megalocornea

Congenital, bilateral, nonprogressive, and symmetrical large corneas with diameters > 13 mm (Fig. 113). Lens subluxation may occur.

Microcornea

Main types
- *True microcornea:* globe has normal dimensions.
- *With sclerocornea:* scleralization of the peripheral cornea, making it appear small.
- *With complex microphthalmos:* globe is also small and variably malformed (Fig. 114).
- *With nanophthalmos:* very hypermetropic eye due to short axial length but otherwise normal.

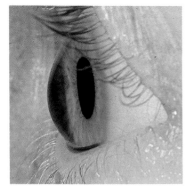

Fig. 109 Keratoconus.

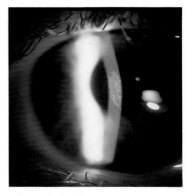

Fig. 110 Vogt's striae.

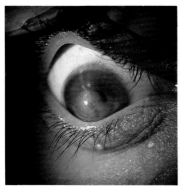

Fig. 111 Acute hydrops and Munson's sign.

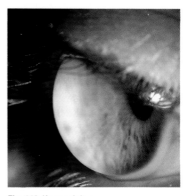

Fig. 112 Keratoglobus.

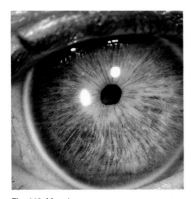

Fig. 113 Megalocornea.

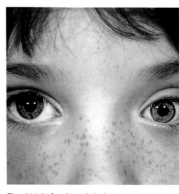

Fig. 114 Left microphthalmos.

Episcleritis
This common and innocuous condition presents with unilateral redness and slight discomfort. The two types are *nodular* (Fig. 115) and *diffuse* (Fig. 116).

Treatment: severe and persistent inflammation requires topical steroids and systemic non-steroidal anti-inflammatory agents.

Scleritis
Causes: Rheumatoid arthritis, Wegener's granulomatosis, polyarteritis nodosa, herpes zoster, surgically-induced, and idiopathic.

Clinical types

Anterior non-necrotizing scleritis
This is the most common type. It may be *nodular* or *diffuse* (Fig. 117).

Anterior necrotizing with inflammation
This is a rare painful condition characterized by local scleral injection and necrosis (Fig. 118). Complications include secondary keratitis, cataract, and glaucoma.

Scleromalacia perforans
This rare condition typically affects patients with seropositive rheumatoid arthritis. It is characterized by painless patches of scleral necrosis unassociated with inflammation that expose the underlying uvea (Fig. 119). Spontaneous perforation is rare but may occur as a result of trauma.

Posterior scleritis
This rare condition may be non-necrotizing or necrotizing with inflammation. The multitude of possible signs includes: proptosis, ophthalmoplegia, disc swelling, macular edema, uveitis, exudative retinal detachment (see Fig. 228), ring choroidal detachment, uveal effusion (Fig. 120), choroidal folds (see Fig. 41), and subretinal exudation.

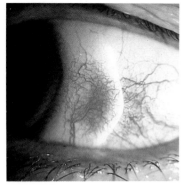

Fig. 115 Nodular episcleritis.

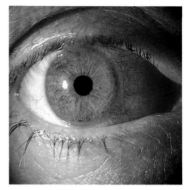

Fig. 116 Diffuse episcleritis.

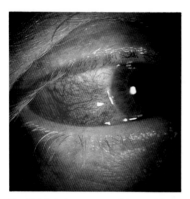

Fig. 117 Anterior non-necrotizing nodular scleritis.

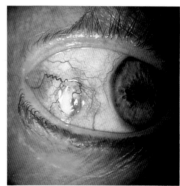

Fig. 118 Anterior necrotizing scleritis with inflammation.

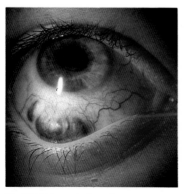

Fig. 119 Scleromalacia perforans.

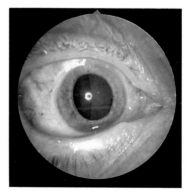

Fig. 120 Uveal effusion.

21 / Anterior uveitis

Etiologic classification

Arthropathies
- HLA-B27-associated (ankylosing spondylitis, Reiter syndrome, psoriatic arthritis, and colitic arthropathy).
- Juvenile rheumatoid arthritis (particularly pauciarticular-onset and positive antinuclear antibody).

Inflammatory bowel disease.

Noninfectious systemic diseases: sarcoidosis, Behçet's, interstitial nephritis, multiple sclerosis, and Vogt–Harada–Koyanagi syndrome.

Infections: syphilis, taberculosis, leprosy, herpes zoster, and herpes simplex.

Idiopathic: Fuchs' uveitis syndrome and sympathetic ophthalmitis.

Clinical features

Symptoms: acute iritis causes a sudden onset of unilateral photophobia, redness, pain, and blurred vision. In chronic anterior uveitis, symptoms may initially be absent or mild.

Signs
- Circumcorneal injection and a small pupil in acute iritis.
- Keratic precipitates (Figs. 121 and 122) may be small in acute iritis or large and mutton fat in granulomatous inflammation.
- Aqueous flare (Fig. 122) and cells.
- Hypopyon (Fig. 123) and a fibrinous exudate.
- Iris nodules in granulomatous inflammation.

Complications
- Posterior synechiae (Fig. 124).
- Band keratopathy and secondary cataract (Fig. 125).
- Secondary glaucoma.
- Iris atrophy (see Fig. 95).
- Phthisis bulb: (Fig. 126) may be the end result of severe chronic uveitis.

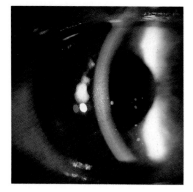

Fig. 121 Keratic precipitates in chronic anterior uveitis.

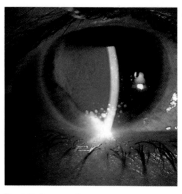

Fig. 122 Aqueous flare and large keratic precipitates.

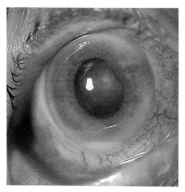

Fig. 123 Hypopyon in severe acute anterior uveitis.

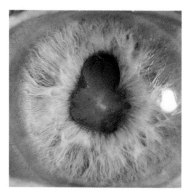

Fig. 124 Adhesions between the lens and iris (posterior synechiae).

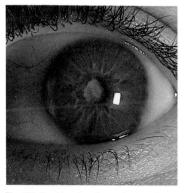

Fig. 125 Band keratopathy and cataract.

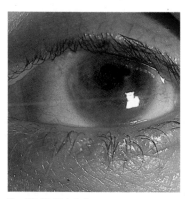

Fig. 126 Phthisis bulb.

Clinical types

Toxoplasmosis
This is caused by reactivation of congenital infection of the protozoan *Toxoplasma gondii*.

Signs: solitary focal retinitis adjacent to an old scar (Fig. 127) associated with vitritis.

Toxocariasis
This is caused by the common intestinal worm of dogs, *Toxocara canis*.

Signs
- *Posterior pole granuloma,* which presents with poor vision between ages 6–14.
- *Peripheral granuloma,* which presents later with distortion of the macula or disc (Fig. 128) or retinal detachment (Fig. 129).
- *Chronic endophthalmitis,* which presents between 2–9 years with leukocoria (see Fig. 235), strabismus (see Fig. 254), or visual loss.

Cytomegalovirus retinitis
This eventually affects 40% of patients with acquired immunodeficency syndrome. Both eyes are involved in 30% of cases.

Signs: starts at the posterior pole with yellow-white areas of retinal necrosis (Fig. 130) associated with variable hemorrhage and mild vitritis. The lesions spread along the vascular arcades (Fig. 131) and cause visual loss as a result of retinal necrosis, optic nerve damage, or retinal detachment.

Presumed ocular histoplasmosis syndrome
This is a fungal infection caused by *Histoplasma capsulatum*.

Signs: punched-out discrete chorioretinal scars usually outside the vascular arcades, peripapillary atrophy (Fig. 132), and neovascular maculopathy. There is no associated vitritis.

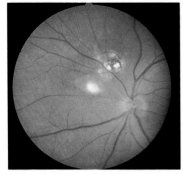

Fig. 127 Active toxoplasmosis.

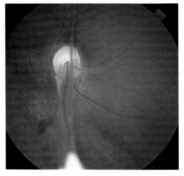

Fig. 128 Peripheral toxocaral granuloma.

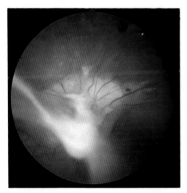

Fig. 129 Large granuloma associated with a retinal detachment in ocular toxocariasis.

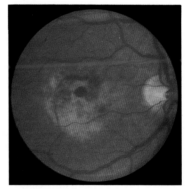

Fig. 130 Central cytomegalovirus retinitis.

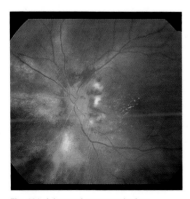

Fig. 131 Advanced cytomegalovirus retinitis.

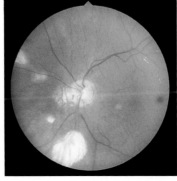

Fig. 132 Chorioretinal atrophy in presumed ocular histoplasmosis syndrome.

Clinical types

Intermediate uveitis

This is a common, idiopathic, insidious, chronic uveitis that typically affects children and young adults. The inflammation predominantly affects the pars plana and the extreme retinal periphery. Both eyes are affected in about 80% of cases.

Signs
- Anterior chamber may show mild activity.
- Vitritis is the most important finding; it may be associated with large focal opacities (Fig. 133).
- Mild peripheral vasculitis.
- Snowbanking of the inferior pars plana may be present in some cases (pars planitis).

Sarcoidosis

This is a multisystem disease characterized by non-caseating granuloma.

Signs
- Periphlebitis—when advanced may give rise to "candlewax drippings" (Fig. 134).
- Retinal granuloma that are typically located inferiorly.
- Choroidal granuloma are bilateral, small, yellow-white lesions (Fig. 135).
- Optic nerve granuloma (Fig. 136) or neovascularization.

Behçet's disease

This is characterized by oral ulceration, recurrent genital ulceration, and skin lesions.

Signs
- Diffuse vascular leakage, which gives rise to chronic retinal edema and cystoid macular edema.
- Periphlebitis, which may result in venous occlusion (Fig. 137).
- Retinitis characterized by white necrotic infiltrates.

Figure 138 shows end-stage diseases with optic atrophy.

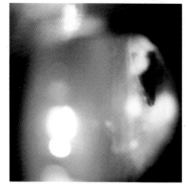

Fig. 133 Severe vitritis in intermediate uveitis.

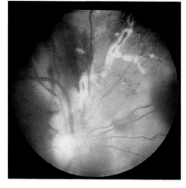

Fig. 134 Retinal vasculitis with "candlewax" perivascular exudates.

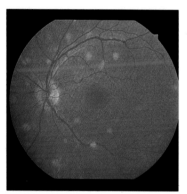

Fig. 135 Sarcoid choroidal granuloma.

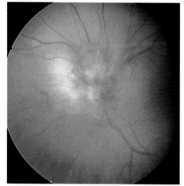

Fig. 136 Optic nerve head sarcoid granuloma.

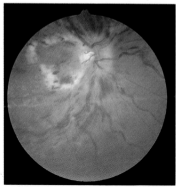

Fig. 137 Severe periphlebitis in Behçet's disease.

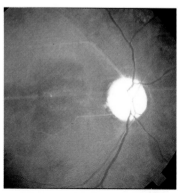

Fig. 138 Optic atrophy in Behçet's disease.

Clinical types

Birdshot retinochoroidopathy

This rare, idiopathic, chronic, bilateral condition typically affects middle-aged women who carry HLA-A29.

Signs
- *Early:* bilateral, multiple, deep, flat creamy yellow spots radiating outward from the disc (Fig. 139) associated with variable vasculitis and vitritis.
- *Late:* circumscribed, atrophic white areas (Fig. 140) that may be associated with cystoid macular edema, vitreous hemorrhage, optic atrophy, and cataract.

Acute posterior multifocal placoid pigment epitheliopathy

This uncommon, idiopathic, acute, bilateral, innocuous condition typically affects young adults.

Signs
- *Early:* deep, placoid, cream-colored lesions (Fig. 141) initially in one eye and then soon after in the other.
- *Late:* after a few weeks, the acute lesions spontaneously disappear, leaving behind diffuse changes involving the retinal pigment epithelium that do not compromise visual acuity (Fig. 142).

Serpiginous choroidopathy

This rare, idiopathic, chronic bilateral condition typically affects middle-aged and elderly adults.

Signs
- *Early:* deep, geographic, cream-colored opacities with hazy borders radiating from the disc. The lesions spread very slowly and gradually coalesce (Fig. 143), but unless the macula is involved, they are asymptomatic.
- *Late:* confluent, scalloped, punched-out atrophic areas that invariably involve the macula (Fig. 144). Subretinal neovascularization occurs in some cases.

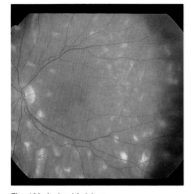

Fig. 139 Active birdshot retinochoroidopathy.

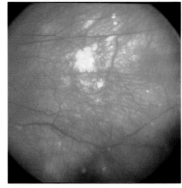

Fig. 140 Inactive birdshot retinochoroidopathy.

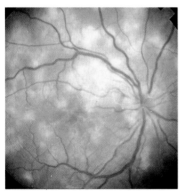

Fig. 141 Active placoid.

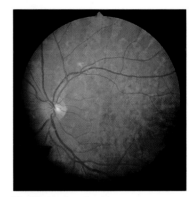

Fig. 142 Inactive placoid.

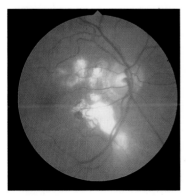

Fig. 143 Active serpiginous choroidopathy.

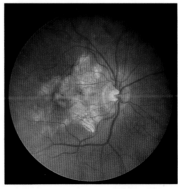

Fig. 144 Extensive macular involvement in serpiginous choroidopathy.

25 / Primary open-angle glaucoma

Definition

Primary open-angle glaucoma (POAG) is a slowly progressive, usually bilateral, disease that affects about 1:200 of the population older than the age of 40 years. Both sexes are affected equally.

Risk factors

- First-degree relatives of patients with POAG; the risk to siblings is approximately 10% and to offspring 4%. It is therefore important to regularly screen first-degree relatives.
- High myopes.
- Steroid responders.
- Patients with retinal vein occlusion.
- Patients with retinitis pigmentosa (see Fig. 217).

Clinical features

Patients are usually asymptomatic until significant loss of visual field has occurred, and frequently the condition is first suspected when a high IOP is detected at a routine eye examination (Fig. 145). Progression of damage is often asymmetrical, so that there may be severe visual field loss in one eye and less advanced disease in the other.

Signs
- The IOP is constantly > 21 mmHg.
- The chamber angle is open and normal.
- Glaucomatous optic nerve damage (Figs. 146–149).
- Characteristic visual field loss.

Treatment

Topical medical therapy
This is usually the initial treatment. One or more of the following drugs may be used.

- *Beta-blockers:* timoptol, betaxolol, levobunolol, carteolol, and metipranolol.
- *Carbonic anhydrase inhibitors:* dorzolamide.
- *Miotics:* pilocarpine and carbachol.
- *Sympathomimetics:* adrenaline and dipivefrin.
- Alpha II agonist.

Laser trabeculoplasty: a useful adjunct to medical therapy.

Trabeculectomy: (filtration surgery—Fig. 150) may be necessary in cases unresponsive to the above measures or as primary treatment for eyes with advanced damage.

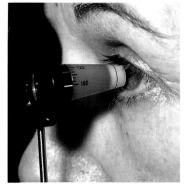

Fig. 145 Measurement of intraocular pressure.

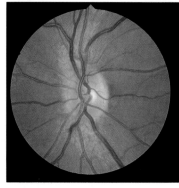

Fig. 146 Normal optic disc.

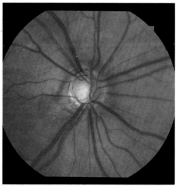

Fig. 147 Early cupping with an inferior notch.

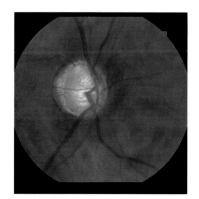

Fig. 148 Moderate cupping.

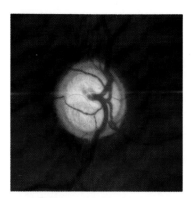

Fig. 149 Advanced cupping.

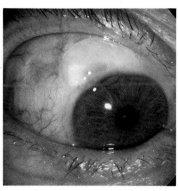

Fig. 150 Conjunctival filtration bleb.

Clinical types

Pigmentary glaucoma
This is caused by blockage of outflow by pigment granules derived from the iris. It typically affects young myopic males.

Signs
- Vertical spindle-shaped area of fine pigment granules on the corneal endothelium (Krukenberg spindle) (Fig. 151).
- Anterior chamber is excessively deep.
- Spoke-like radial defects in the mid-peripheral iris.
- Pigment granules on the anterior iris surface.
- Trabecular hyperpigmentation (Fig. 152).

Pseudoexfoliation glaucoma
This is caused by blockage of outflow by pseudoexfoliative material. It typically affects the elderly.

Signs
- Pseudoexfoliative material on the anterior lens surface (Fig. 153) and pupillary border (Fig. 154).
- Trabecular hyperpigmentation and "dandruff-like" deposits of pseudoexfoliative material.
- Atrophy of sphincter pupillae.

Post-traumatic angle recession glaucoma
This is caused by blunt traumatic trabecular damage. Elevation of IOP usually occurs months or years after the initial injury.

Signs
- Signs of previous damage such as tears in the iris sphincter or iridodialysis (see Fig. 268).
- The angle is irregular, scarred, and recessed (Fig. 155).

Phacolytic glaucoma
This is a unilateral acute trabecular block glaucoma associated with a hypermature cataract.

Signs: deep anterior chamber; aqueous may contain floating white particles (Fig. 156).

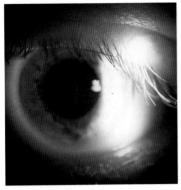

Fig. 151 Krukenberg spindle in pigmentary glaucoma.

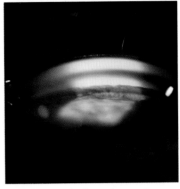

Fig. 152 Trabecular hyperpigmentation.

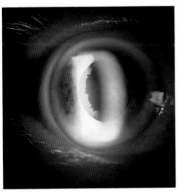

Fig. 153 Pseudoexfoliation of the anterior lens capsule.

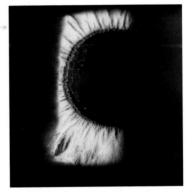

Fig. 154 Pseudoexfoliative material on lens and pupillary border.

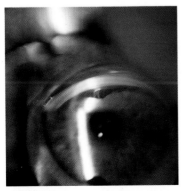

Fig. 155 Severe angle recession.

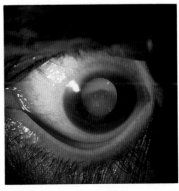

Fig. 156 Hypermature cataract.

Definition

Primary angle-closure glaucoma is a condition in which elevation of IOP occurs as a result of obstruction to aqueous outflow.

Risk factors

- Age older than 60 years and female.
- Positive family history.
- Shallow anterior chamber and narrow angle.
- Hypermetropia.

Clinical types

Subacute angle-closure glaucoma
This is caused by intermittent angle closure. Symptoms are transient blurring of vision and halos around lights associated with eye ache. In between attacks, the eye looks normal.

Treatment: laser iridotomy (Fig. 157).

Acute angle-closure glaucoma
This is caused by a sudden total occlusion of the angle (Fig. 158). Symptoms include an acute loss of vision associated with ocular pain and occasionally nausea and vomiting.

Signs
- Very high IOP.
- Circumcorneal "ciliary" injection.
- Corneal epithelial edema (Fig. 159).
- Peripheral iridocorneal contact.
- Pupil is fixed, oval, and semidilated (Fig. 160).

Treatment
- Systemic carbonic anhydrase inhibitors and, if necessary, hyperosmotic agents.
- Topical miotics, beta-blockers, and steroids.
- Laser iridotomy once the IOP has been reduced.

Chronic sign angle-closure glaucoma

Signs
- Stromal iris atrophy with a spiral-like configuration and fine pigment granules on its surface (Fig. 161).
- Fixed and semidilated pupil.
- Aqueous flare and cells.
- Anterior lens opacity (glaukomflecken—Fig. 162).

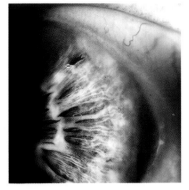

Fig. 157 Laser iridotomy.

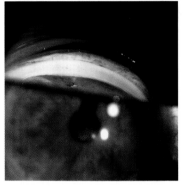

Fig. 158 Total angle closure.

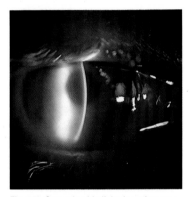

Fig. 159 Corneal epithelial edema in acute angle-closure glaucoma.

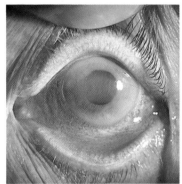

Fig. 160 Fixed and dilated pupil in acute angle-closure glaucoma.

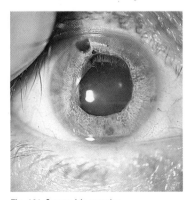

Fig. 161 Severe iris atrophy.

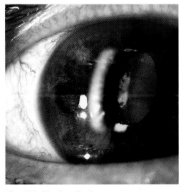

Fig. 162 Glaukomflecken.

Clinical types

Neovascular glaucoma

This common and very serious condition is caused by synechial angle closure by contraction of fibrovascular tissue. By far the most important cause is diabetes.

Signs
- Usually very high IOP and corneal edema.
- A painful and congested globe.
- Very poor visual acuity.
- Aqueous flare.
- Severe rubeosis iridis, pupillary distortion, and ectropion uveae (Figs. 163 and 164).

Iridocorneal endothelial syndrome

This causes synechial angle closure glaucoma by contraction of abnormal corneal endothelial cells.

Types
- *Progressive iris atrophy:* stromal atrophy, hole formation and corectopia (Figs. 165 and 166).
- *Iris nevus (Cogan–Reese) syndrome:* either diffuse iris nevus or pigmented pedunculated iris nodules.
- *Chandler syndrome:* severe corneal endothelial changes.

Treatment: artificial filtrating shunts are usually required (Fig. 167).

Inflammatory angle-closure glaucomas

Mechanisms
- With pupil block secondary to 360° posterior synechiae. It is characterized by a shallow anterior chamber associated with seclusio pupillae and iris bombè (Fig. 168).
- Without pupil block that is caused by contraction of inflammatory debris in the angle and the formation of peripheral anterior synechiae.

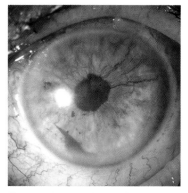

Fig. 163 Advanced rubeosis iridis.

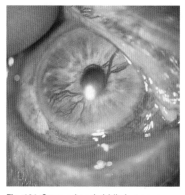

Fig. 164 Gross rubeosis iridis in an eye with advanced neovascular glaucoma.

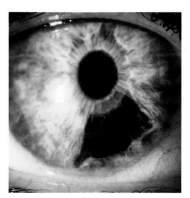

Fig. 165 Progressive iris atrophy.

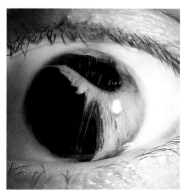

Fig. 166 Very advanced progressive iris atrophy.

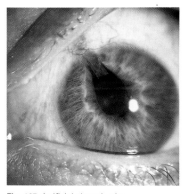

Fig. 167 Artificial shunt in situ.

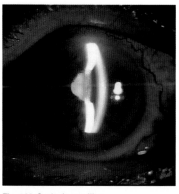

Fig. 168 Seclusio pupillae.

Definition

The congenital glaucomas are a diverse group of rare conditions in which a congenital angle anomaly is responsible for raised IOP.

Primary congenital glaucoma

Clinical types

This condition affects 1 in 10,000 live births.

Signs
- Large eye (buphthalmos, Fig. 169) if the IOP becomes elevated before age 3 years.
- Breaks in Descemet's membrane (Fig. 170).
- Specific angle anomalies.

Rieger anomaly

This may cause secondary angle-closure glaucoma during early childhood.

Signs
- Posterior embryotoxon associated with extensive peripheral anterior synechiae (Fig. 171).
- Iris hypoplasia, holes, ectropion uveae, and corectopia (Fig. 172).

Aniridia

This may cause glaucoma during late childhood due to secondary angle closure by rudimentary iris tissue. The aniridia may be complete or partial (Fig. 173). The three phenotypes are
- AN-1 (85%): isolated ocular defect (autosomal dominant)
- AN-2 (13%): Wilms tumor, genitourinary anomalies, and mental handicap. Associated with deletion of short arm of chromosome 11 (Miller syndrome)
- AN-3 (2%): mental handicap and cerebellar ataxia (autosomal recessive)

Phacomatoses
- *Sturge–Weber syndrome* (Fig. 174) is associated with glaucoma in 30% of cases.
- *Neurofibromatosis type 1* is occasionally associated with glaucoma.

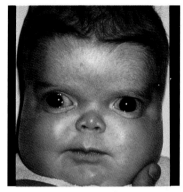

Fig. 169 Bilateral buphthalmos.

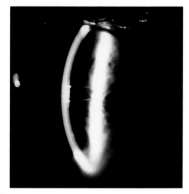

Fig. 170 Breaks in Descemet's membrane in primary congenital glaucoma.

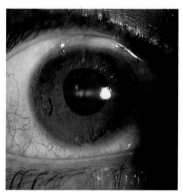

Fig. 171 Rieger anomaly with anterior synechiae and iris hypoplasia.

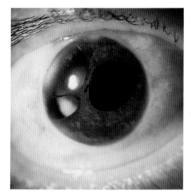

Fig. 172 Large defects in the iris in advanced Rieger anomaly.

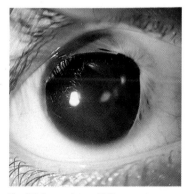

Fig. 173 Incomplete aniridia.

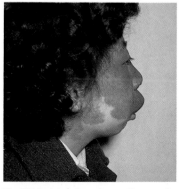

Fig. 174 Facial angioma (nevus flammeus).

Classifications

According to clinical types
- *Subcapsular cataract* may be anterior or posterior (Fig. 175). Patients characteristically have more problems with reading than distance vision.
- *Nuclear cataract* (Fig. 176) initially causes an increase in myopia so that distance vision is affected more than near vision.
- *Cortical cataract* is characterized by spoke-like opacities that can be detected against a red reflex (Fig. 177).

According to state of maturity
- *Immature cataract,* in which there are clear zones between the opacities (see Fig. 177).
- *Mature cataract,* in which the whole lens is opaque and the pupil white (Fig. 178).
- *Hypermature cataract,* which is a shrunken mature cataract with a wrinkled capsule. Eyes with hypermature cataracts may develop phacolytic glaucoma (see Fig. 156).
- *Morgagnian cataract,* which is a hypermature cataract with liquefied cortex and an inferior subluxation of the nucleus.

Surgery

The cataract is removed, and the crystalline lens is replaced by an artificial intraocular lens implant (Fig. 179). There are two surgical techniques.

- *Extracapsular extraction*, which involves a large incision, removal of part of the anterior capsule, expression of the nucleus, and aspiration of residual cortical material.
- *Phacoemulsification,* in which the nucleus and cortex are removed through a small incision by using a special probe.

Capsular opacification eventually occurs in about 20% of cases (Fig. 180).

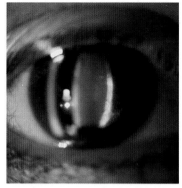

Fig. 175 Posterior subcapsular cataract.

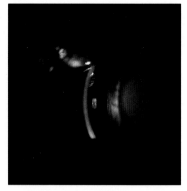

Fig. 176 Nuclear age-related cataract.

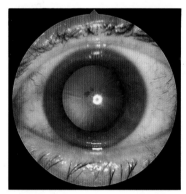

Fig. 177 Cortical cataract seen against the red reflex.

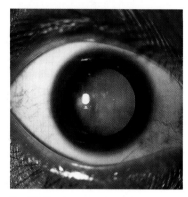

Fig. 178 Nearly mature cataract.

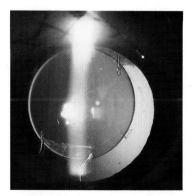

Fig. 179 Posterior chamber intraocular lens implant.

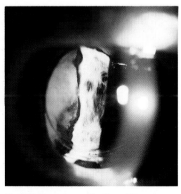

Fig. 180 Severe opacification of the posterior capsule.

Secondary cataract

The opacities are usually posterior (see Fig. 175).

Causes
- *Trauma.*
- *Ocular disease:* chronic iridocyclitis (see Fig. 125), high myopia, and acute glaucoma (see Fig. 162).
- *Systemic diseases:* diabetes, myotonic dystrophy (see Fig. 30), and atopic dermatitis (see Fig. 1).
- *Drug induced:* strong miotics, steroids (systemic and topical), busulfan, and chlorpromazine.

Infantile cataract

The opacity has various shapes (Figs. 181 & 182).

Causes
- *Idiopathic sporadic:* may be unilateral.
- *Hereditary:* most frequently autosomal dominant.
- *Other ocular malformations:* persistent hyperplastic primary vitreous, retinopathy of prematurity, and aniridia (see Fig. 173).
- *Embryopathies:* intrauterine infections such as rubella, toxoplasmosis, and cytomegalovirus.
- *Metabolic:* galactokinase deficiency, galactosemia, and hypocalcemia.
- *Syndromes:* Lowe, Down, Turner, cri-du-chat, Werner, Cockayne, and Rothmund–Thomson.

Ectopia lentis

Causes
- *Blunt ocular trauma* (Fig. 183).
- *Familial ectopia lentis,* which may be associated with ectopic pupil (Fig. 184).
- *Syndromes:* Marfan (Fig. 185), Weill–Marchesani, Ehlers–Danlos, and Stickler.
- *Metabolic:* homocystinuria, hyperlysinemia, and sulfite oxidase deficiency.

Abnormalities of lens size and shape

Clinical types
- *Microphakia* (small lens) in Lowe syndrome.
- *Microspherophakia* (small spherical lens) in Marfan syndrome, Weill–Marchesani syndrome, and hyperlysinemia.
- *Coloboma* (Fig. 186).
- *Posterior lenticonus*.
- *Anterior lenticonus* in Alport syndrome.

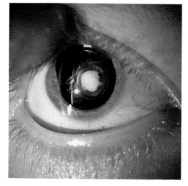

Fig. 181 Nuclear congenital cataract.

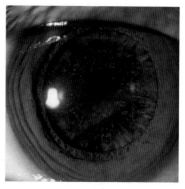

Fig. 182 Punctate congenital lens opacities.

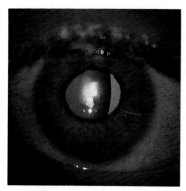

Fig. 183 Lens subluxation due to blunt ocular trauma.

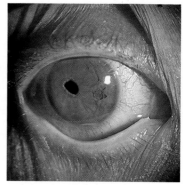

Fig. 184 Congenital ectopic pupil associated with lens subluxation.

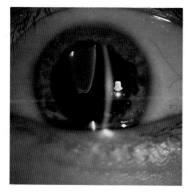

Fig. 185 Upward lens subluxation in Marfan syndrome.

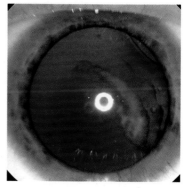

Fig. 186 Lens coloboma and opacity.

Diabetic retinopathy (DR) is the most common cause of blindness in the 30–60 age group. The incidence of DR is related primarily to the duration of diabetes.

Clinical types

Background diabetic retinopathy

This is characterized by microaneurysms, deep dot and blot hemorrhages, retinal edema, and hard exudates (Fig. 187). Visual acuity is normal, and apart from regular fundus examination, treatment is unnecessary.

Diabetic maculopathies

Maculopathy is the most common cause of visual impairment in patients with diabetes. The three main types are

- *Focal maculopathy,* caused by the spillover of edema and/or hard exudates into the fovea from leaking microaneurysms (Fig. 188).
- *Diffuse maculopathy,* caused by extensive leakage.
- *Ischemic maculopathy.*

Preproliferative diabetic retinopathy

This is characterized by cotton wool spots (Fig. 189), intraretinal microvascular anomalies, venous changes (dilation, beading, looping, and sausage-like segmentation—Fig. 190), arteriolar narrowing, and large dark blot hemorrhages.

Proliferative diabetic retinopathy

This is characterized by neovascularization of the disc (Figs. 190 and 191) and/or the retina (Fig. 192). The new vessels may be flat or elevated, and they may be associated with variable amounts of fibrous tissue. Unless treated, severe visual loss may occur as a result of vitreous hemorrhage and tractional retinal detachment (see Fig. 227).

Treatment

- *Laser photocoagulation* for focal and diffuse maculopathy and proliferative retinopathy.
- *Vitrectomy* for persistent vitreous hemorrhage and tractional retinal detachment involving the macula.

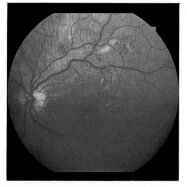

Fig. 187 Mild background retinopathy.

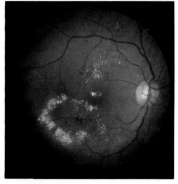

Fig. 188 Severe background retinopathy.

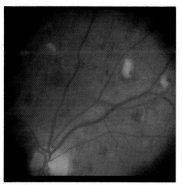

Fig. 189 Cotton wool spots.

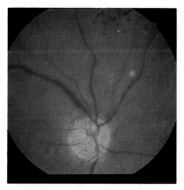

Fig. 190 Severe venous changes and mild disc new vessels with a few laser scars.

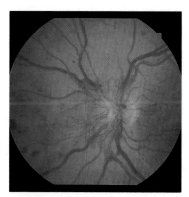

Fig. 191 Severe proliferative diabetic retinopathy.

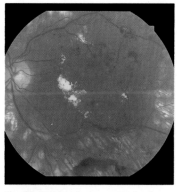

Fig. 192 Peripheral new vessels, hard exudates, and laser scars.

Clinical types

Retinal vein occlusion

Predisposing factors: systemic hypertension and arteriosclerosis, raised IOP, blood hyperviscosity, and retinal periphlebitis.

Signs
- *Early:* venous changes, hemorrhages, disc edema, retinal edema, and cotton wool spots.
- *Late:* venous sheathing, collaterals, and hard exudates (Fig. 193).

Classification
- *Branch vein occlusion* (Fig. 194).
- *Hemisphere vein occlusion* (Fig. 195).
- *Central vein occlusion* (Fig. 196).

Complications
- *Neovascularization,* particularly retinal, is a common complication of branch retinal vein occlusion.
- *Chronic macular edema* may occur in all types of occlusion.
- *Neovascular glaucoma,* mainly seen in central retinal vein occlusion (see Fig. 163).

Retinal artery occlusion

Causes: vaso-obliteration by atheroma or arteritis, and embolization.

Presentation: acute loss of vision which may be permanent or transient (amaurosis fugax).

Signs
Arteriolar narrowing, segmentation of the blood column (cattle-trucking), and retinal pallor (Fig. 197). In central retinal artery occlusion, a "cherry red spot" at the fovea is seen (Fig. 198).

Treatment
- *Amaurosis fugax:* aspirin or carotid endarterectomy if severe carotid stenosis is present.
- *Acute permanent obstruction:* intermittent ocular massage, intravenous injection of 500 mg acetazolamide, and paracentesis of the anterior chamber.

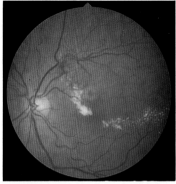

Fig. 193 Collaterals and hard exudates in old venous occlusion.

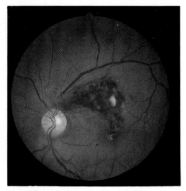

Fig. 194 Acute branch retinal vein occlusion.

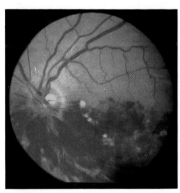

Fig. 195 Acute inferior hemisphere retinal vein occlusion.

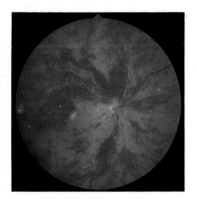

Fig. 196 Central retinal vein occlusion.

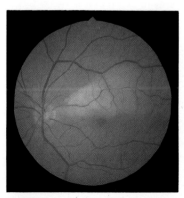

Fig. 197 Acute branch retinal artery occlusion.

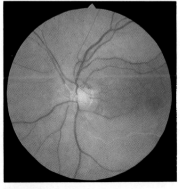

Fig. 198 Acute central retinal artery occlusion.

Clinical types

Hypertensive retinopathy

Grading
- *Grade 1:* mild generalized arteriolar constriction, broadening of the arteriolar light reflex, and vein concealment (Fig. 199).
- *Grade 2:* severe arteriolar constriction associated with deflection of veins at arteriovenous crossings (Salus' sign) (Fig. 200).
- *Grade 3:* copper wiring of arterioles associated with severe venous changes at arteriovenous crossings such as banking (Bonnet's sign), tapering (Gunn's sign), and right-angled deflections. Other features include flame-shaped hemorrhages, cotton wool spots, and hard exudates (Fig. 201).
- *Grade 4:* silver wiring of arterioles and disc swelling (Fig. 202).

Proliferative sickle cell retinopathy

Stages
- *Stage 1:* peripheral arteriolar occlusion.
- *Stage 2:* peripheral arteriovenous anastamoses.
- *Stage 3:* sprouting of new vessels from anastamoses.
- *Stage 4:* vitreous hemorrhage (Fig. 203).
- *Stage 5:* tractional retinal detachment.

Retinopathy of prematurity
This affects preterm infants exposed to high ambient levels of oxygen.

Stages of active disease
- *Stage 1:* demarcation mark parallel to the ora serrata.
- *Stage 2:* ridge with isolated neovascular tufts.
- *Stage 3:* ridge with extraretinal fibrovascular proliferation associated with dilated and tortuous vessels (Fig. 204).
- *Stage 4:* subtotal tractional retinal detachment.
- *Stage 5:* total retinal detachment.

"Plus" disease is characterized by iris congestion and rigidity, venous dilation, and arteriolar tortuosity in the posterior fundus.

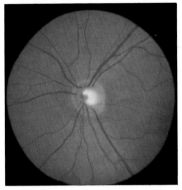

Fig. 199 Generalized arteriolar constriction in grade 1 hypertensive retinopathy.

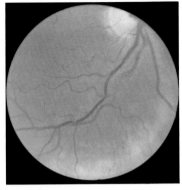

Fig. 200 Focal arteriolar constriction in grade 2 hypertensive retinopathy.

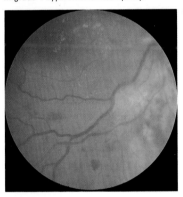

Fig. 201 Severe arteriovenous changes, hemorrhages, and exudates in grade 3 hypertensive retinopathy.

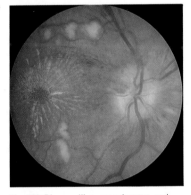

Fig. 202 Disc swelling, macular star, and cotton wool spots in grade 4 hypertensive retinopathy.

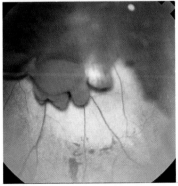

Fig. 203 Vitreous hemorrhage in stage 4 sickle cell retinopathy.

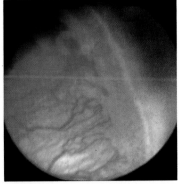

Fig. 204 Ridge with fibrovascular proliferation in stage 3 retinopathy.

Age-related macular degeneration (AMD) typically affects patients older than the age of 65 years and eventually usually affects both eyes.

Clinical features

Drusen

Drusen (colloid bodies) are bilateral, yellow-white, slightly elevated spots at the posterior pole.

- *Hard drusen* are small, round, and discrete. They are usually innocuous.
- *Soft drusen* are larger and have ill-defined edges (Fig. 205) and are associated with AMD.

Nonexudative macular degeneration

This causes a slowly progressive loss of central vision.

Signs
- *Early:* pigmentary changes involving the retinal pigment epithelium (RPE) followed by the development of sharply circumscribed circular areas of atrophy of the RPE.
- *Late:* larger choroidal vessels become prominent within the atrophic areas (Fig. 206).

Exudative macular degeneration

Presentation is with a subacute onset of unilateral distortion of central vision.

Signs
- *Hemorrhagic RPE detachment* due to bleeding from a neovascular membrane.
- *Hemorrhagic detachment of the sensory retina* (Fig. 207).
- *Subretinal scarring* (Figs. 208 and 209).
- *Extensive subretinal exudation* (Fig. 210) occurs in some eyes.

Treatment: laser photocoagulation aimed at destroying the subretinal neovascular membranes may be beneficial in a few carefully selected early cases. Patients with permanent loss of central vision may benefit from special magnifying (low vision) aids.

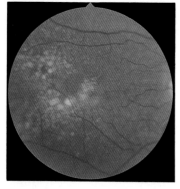

Fig. 205 Macular drusen (colloid bodies).

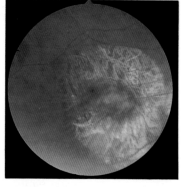

Fig. 206 Advanced geographic atrophy.

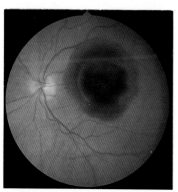

Fig. 207 Subretinal hemorrhage.

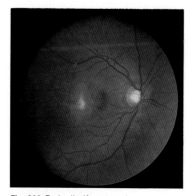

Fig. 208 Early disciform scarring.

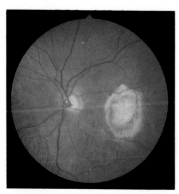

Fig. 209 Advanced disciform scarring.

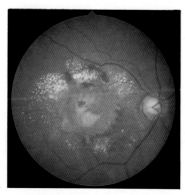

Fig. 210 Subretinal exudation.

Clinical types

Age-related macular hole

Signs: round "punched-out" area at the fovea surrounded by a gray halo of retinal elevation (Fig. 211).

Myopic maculopathy

Signs
- *Early:* atrophy of the RPE and choriocapillaris with unmasking of the large choroidal vessels.
- *Late:* proliferation of the RPE at the fovea (Fuchs' spot—Fig. 212), breaks in Bruch's membrane (lacquer cracks), atrophic maculopathy (Fig. 213), and macular hemorrhage.

Macular pucker

Causes: retinal vascular disease, trauma, retinal surgery, retinal photocoagulation or cryotherapy, and chronic intraocular inflammation. In elderly patients, the condition is frequently idiopathic.

Signs
- *Early* (cellophane maculopathy): translucent epiretinal membrane associated with mild retinal wrinkling and vascular tortuosity.
- *Late:* opaque epiretinal membrane associated with marked vascular tortuosity (Fig. 214).

Angioid streaks
These are associated with pseudoxanthoma elasticum in about 50% of patients.

Signs: bilateral linear streaks radiating from the disc (Fig. 215). Maculopathy may be caused by a streak, choroidal neovascularization, or traumatic subfoveal hemorrhage.

Bull's eye maculopathy

Causes: antimalarials, cone dystrophy, Stargardt's disease (see Fig. 218), and Batten's disease.

Signs: central foveolar hyperpigmentation surrounded by a depigmented zone that is encircled by a hyperpigmented ring (Fig. 216).

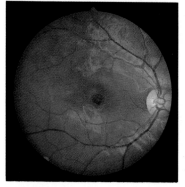

Fig. 211 Macular hole.

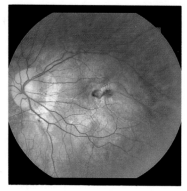

Fig. 212 Fuchs' spot in myopia.

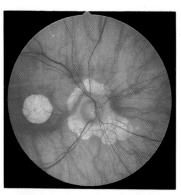

Fig. 213 Atrophic myopic maculopathy.

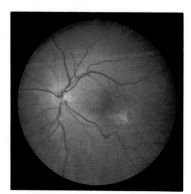

Fig. 214 Macular pucker.

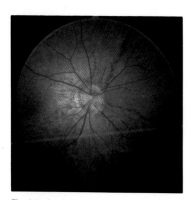

Fig. 215 Angioid streaks.

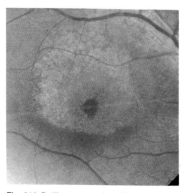

Fig. 216 Bull's eye maculopathy.

Clinical types

Retinitis pigmentosa
Presentation is during the second decade of life with night blindness.

Signs: mid-peripheral perivascular "bone-spicule" pigmentation, arteriolar attenuation, unmasking of large choroidal vessels, and waxy disc pallor (Fig. 217).

Associated systemic syndromes: Bassen–Kornzweig, Refsum, Usher, Cockayne, Kearns–Sayre, Bardet–Biedl, and Laurence–Moon.

Stargardt's macular dystrophy
Presentation of this is between the first and second decades, with gradual asymmetrical impairment of visual acuity.

Signs: "snail-slime" oval macular lesion that may later assume an atrophic "bull's eye" configuration (Fig. 218).

Fundus flavimaculatus
Presentation is during the fourth or fifth decade.

Signs: ill-defined, yellow-white flecks or spots (Fig. 219). Later maculopathy similar to Stargardt's may develop.

Best's disease

Stages
- *Vitelliform:* egg yolk macular lesion (Fig. 220).
- *Pseudohypyon:* partial absorption of the lesion.
- *Vitelliruptive:* "scrambled egg" appearance.
- *End-stage:* macular scar.

Choroidal dystrophies
- *Choroideremia:* enlarging midretinal patches of chorioretinal atrophy that progressively spread centrally but spare the macula until late (Fig. 221).
- *Gyrate atrophy:* coalescing midretinal patches of chorioretinal atrophy (Fig. 222).

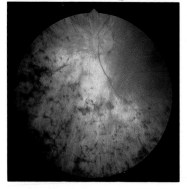

Fig. 217 Retinitis pigmentosa.

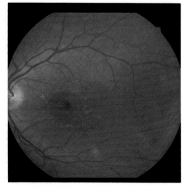

Fig. 218 Stargardt's dystrophy.

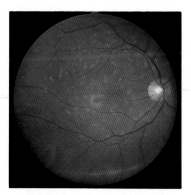

Fig. 219 Fundus flavimaculatus.

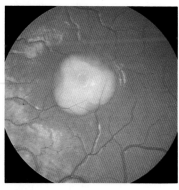

Fig. 220 "Egg yolk" stage of Best's disease.

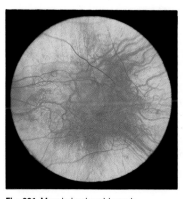

Fig. 221 Macula in choroideremia.

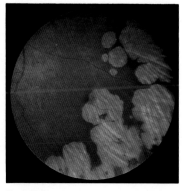

Fig. 222 Gyrate atrophy.

Definition

A retinal detachment (RD) is a separation of the neuroretina from the underlying RPE by the accumulation of subretinal fluid (SRF).

Clinical types

Rhegmatogenous retinal detachment

Cause: retinal break (Fig. 223) developing as a result of interplay between vitreoretinal traction and a weakness in the peripheral retina, most frequently lattice degeneration (Fig. 224).

Signs
- *Fresh RD:* mobile, convex, and corrugated appearance with loss of the underlying choroidal pattern (Fig. 225).
- *Long-standing RD:* retinal thinning, secondary cysts, and demarcation lines (high-water marks).
- *Proliferative vitreoretinopathy:* fibrotic and immobile retina (Fig. 226).

Treatment
- Scleral buckling for uncomplicated cases.
- Vitrectomy for complicated cases.

Tractional retinal detachment

Causes: progressive pulling on the retina by contraction of fibrous or fibrovascular membranes.

Signs: concave immobile RD with shallow SRF that seldom extends to the ora serrata (Fig. 227).

Treatment: by pars plana vitrectomy if the macula is threatened.

Exudative retinal detachment
- *Intraocular tumors.*
- *Intraocular inflammation.*
- *Severe leakage from subretinal neovascular membranes* (see Fig. 210).
- *Iatrogenic:* after retinal surgery and panretinal photocoagulation (see Fig. 192).
- *Severe hypertension.*

Signs: convex and very mobile RD, which may be associated with subretinal pigment clumping (Fig. 228).

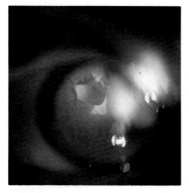

Fig. 223 Large retinal tear.

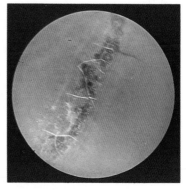

Fig. 224 Lattice degeneration.

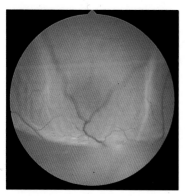

Fig. 225 Superior rhegmatogenous RD.

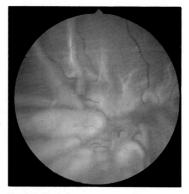

Fig. 226 Total rhegmatogenous RD complicated by severe fibrosis.

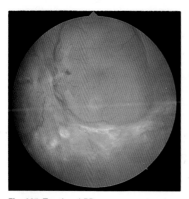

Fig. 227 Tractional RD.

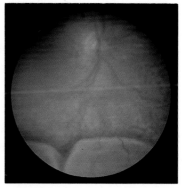

Fig. 228 Exudative RD with "leopard spots".

Clinical types

Choroidal melanoma

This is the most common malignant intraocular tumor in adults.

Signs: brown, black, or amelanotic oval-shaped mass (Fig. 229). Associated features include secondary exudative retinal detachment, surface orange lipofuscin pigment, choroidal folds, and intraocular inflammation.

Iris melanoma

Signs: pigmented or nonpigmented inferior iris nodule (Fig. 230). Associated features include ectropion uveae, iris neovascularization, pupillary distortion, cataract, and raised IOP.

Choroidal nevus

This common benign tumor is usually found by chance.

Signs: flat or slightly elevated, oval or round slate-gray lesion that is usually < 3 mm in diameter, which may be associated with surface drusen (Fig. 231).

Localized choroidal hemangioma

Signs: dome-shaped or placoid, orange-red lesion that is typically located at the posterior pole (Fig. 232). It may be associated with secondary cystoid degeneration and pigment mottling. Pressure on the globe may induce blanching of the tumor.

Metastatic choroidal carcinoma

Signs: solitary or multiple, unilateral or bilateral, creamy white oval lesions with ill-defined borders, most commonly located at the posterior pole (Fig. 233).

Choroidal osteoma

Signs: usually unilateral, slightly elevated, orange-yellow lesion with geographic and well-demarcated borders at the posterior pole (Fig. 234).

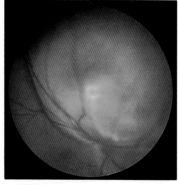

Fig. 229 Large melanoma of the choroid.

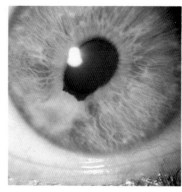

Fig. 230 Melanoma of the iris.

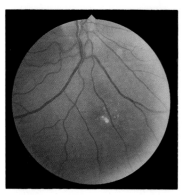

Fig. 231 Choroidal nevus with overlying drusen.

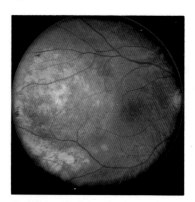

Fig. 232 Localized choroidal hemangioma.

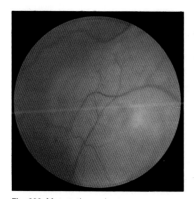

Fig. 233 Metastatic carcinoma.

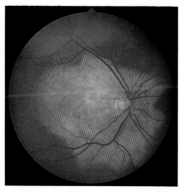

Fig. 234 Choroidal osteoma.

Clinical types

Retinoblastoma

This is the most common malignant intraocular tumor in children. It is bilateral in 30% of cases.

Presentation: usually at about 18 months with a white pupil (leukocoria) (Fig. 235). Other presentations include strabismus, secondary glaucoma, and anterior chamber infiltration.

Signs
- *Endophytic tumor:* grows into the vitreous cavity and appears as a white mass with fine surface blood vessels.
- *Exophytic tumor:* grows in the subretinal space and causes a retinal detachment.

Retinal astrocytoma

This typically affects patients with tuberous sclerosis.

Signs: whitish round mass that is frequently situated near the optic nerve head (Fig. 236).

Retinal capillary hemangioma

This is frequently multiple, and both eyes are affected in 50% of cases. 25% of patients also have the von Hippel–Lindau syndrome.

Signs: round orange-red lesion that is associated with marked dilation of the supplying artery and draining vein (Fig. 237).

Retinal cavernous hemangioma

Signs: grape-like saccular aneurysms filled with dark blood (Fig. 238).

Retinal racemose hemangioma

This may be associated with the Wyburn–Mason syndrome.

Signs: grossly dilated and tortuous vessels (Fig. 239).

Melanocytoma of the optic nerve head

Signs: black lesion with feathery edges (Fig. 240).

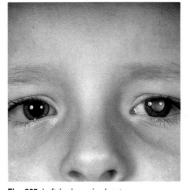

Fig. 235 Left leukocoria due to retinoblastoma.

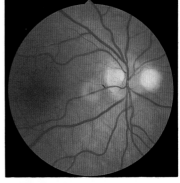

Fig. 236 Retinal astrocytoma.

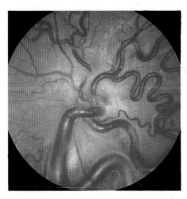

Fig. 237 Capillary hemangioma.

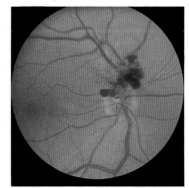

Fig. 238 Cavernous hemangioma.

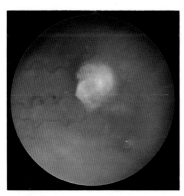

Fig. 239 Racemose hemangioma.

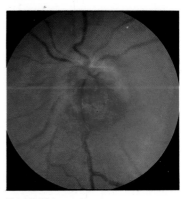

Fig. 240 Melanocytoma.

Clinical types

Optic neuritis
This is an inflammatory or demyelinating disorder of the optic nerve.

Main types
- *Retrobulbar neuritis:* normal fundus. This is most common in adults and is frequently associated with multiple sclerosis. Severe or recurrent attacks may result in optic atrophy (Fig. 241).
- *Papillitis:* disc swelling and vitreous cells. This is most common in children and may be bilateral.
- *Neuroretinitis:* papillitis and a macular star (Fig. 242). This is the least common and is not associated with multiple sclerosis.

Anterior ischemic optic neuropathy
This is an infarction of the optic nerve head.

Main types
- *Arteritic* is associated with giant cell arteritis.
- *Nonarteritic* is associated with hypertension.

Signs: pale and swollen disc that may be associated with splinter-shaped hemorrhages (Fig. 243).

Papilledema
This is bilateral disc swelling caused by raised intracranial pressure.

Signs
- *Early:* disc hyperemia and indistinct margins (Fig. 244).
- *Established:* dilated veins and peripapillary hemorrhages (Fig. 245).
- *Long-standing:* grossly dilated veins, hemorrhages, disc elevation, and hard exudates (Fig. 246).

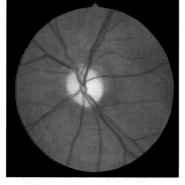

Fig. 241 Optic atrophy.

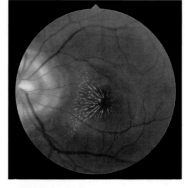

Fig. 242 Neuroretinitis.

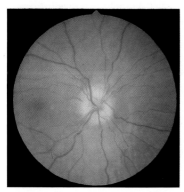

Fig. 243 Arteritic anterior ischemic optic neuropathy.

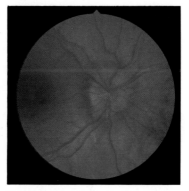

Fig. 244 Early papilledema with indistinct disc margins.

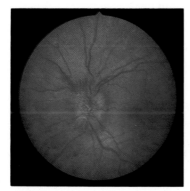

Fig. 245 Established papilledema with flame-shaped hemorrhages.

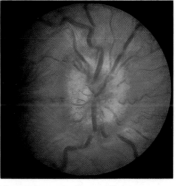

Fig. 246 Long-standing papilledema.

Clincial types

Optic disc drusen

These uncommon lesions are composed of hyaline-like calcific material within the optic nerve head. They are often bilateral and familial.

Signs: elevated optic nerve head with a pink or yellowish color and no physiologic cup. The disc margins are lumpy, and emerging blood vessels have anomalous branching (Fig. 247). During the second decade of life, the drusen usually emerge to the surface of the disc as pearl-like irregularities.

Tilted disc

Signs: oval disc with its vertical axis directed obliquely (Fig. 248). Associated findings include inferior crescent, situs inversus, myopia, and astigmatism. Ectasia of the inferonasal fundus may give rise to an upper temporal visual field defect.

Myelinated nerve fibers

Signs: white feathery-shaped patches that may be mistaken for papilledema when located around the optic disc (Fig. 249).

Optic disc pit

Signs: dark round or oval pit in a larger-than-normal disc (Fig. 250). About 50% of eyes develop a serous detachment of the macula.

Optic disc coloboma

Signs: large inferior excavation that may mimic advanced glaucomatous cupping (Fig. 251). Visual acuity is usually impaired, and a superior visual field defect is present.

Morning glory anomaly

Signs: enlarged and excavated optic nerve head with hyaloid remnants within its base and radially emerging blood vessels (Fig. 252). Visual acuity is poor.

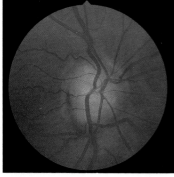

Fig. 247 Optic disc drusen (hyaline bodies).

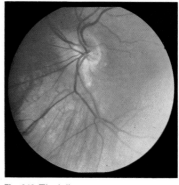

Fig. 248 Tilted disc.

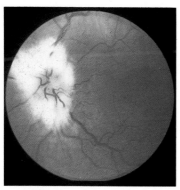

Fig. 249 Myelinated nerve fibers.

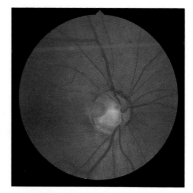

Fig. 250 Optic disc pit.

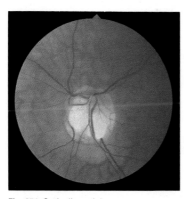

Fig. 251 Optic disc coloboma.

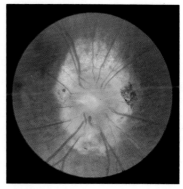

Fig. 252 Morning glory anomaly.

Clinical types

Infantile convergent squint (esotropia)
Presentation is at about or before 6 months of age. It should not be confused with a pseudoesotropia associated with epicanthic folds (Fig. 253).

Signs
- Large and constant angle (Fig. 254).
- Occasionally inferior oblique overaction.

Accommodative esotropia
Presentation is typically at about 2.5 years.

Types
- *Refractive,* caused by excessive hypermetropia.
- *Nonrefractive,* caused by a high AC/A ratio.
- *Mixed,* caused by a combination of both.

Nonaccommodative esotropia
- *Secondary,* caused by a monocular organic lesion that interferes with vision.
- *Consecutive,* caused by excessive surgery.

Divergent squint (exotropia)

Types
- *Congenital.*
- *Decompensating intermittent* (Fig. 255).
- *Secondary,* similar to esotropic counterpart.
- *Consecutive,* caused by excessive surgery.

Duane retraction syndrome

Signs
- Usually straight eyes in the primary position.
- Abduction severely restricted (Fig. 256).
- Retraction of the globe and narrowing of the palpebral fissure on adduction (Fig. 257).

Brown syndrome

Signs
- Straight eyes in the primary position.
- Limited elevation in adduction (Fig. 258).

Management
- Examination of the fundus and refraction.
- Correction of significant refractive errors.
- Treatment of amblyopia by occlusion.
- Surgery to straighten the eyes if appropriate.

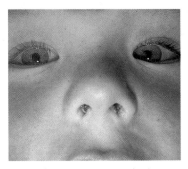

Fig. 253 Pseudoconvergent squint due to epicanthic folds. Note symmetrical corneal reflexes.

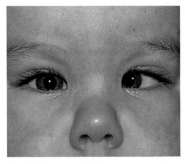

Fig. 254 Congenital left convergent squint. Note asymmetrical corneal reflexes.

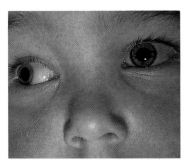

Fig. 255 Right divergent squint.

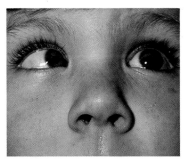

Fig. 256 Left Duane syndrome in abduction.

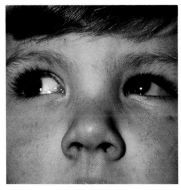

Fig. 257 Left Duane syndrome in adduction.

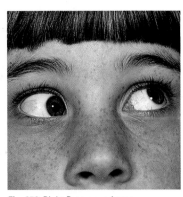

Fig. 258 Right Brown syndrome.

Clinical features

Third nerve palsy

Signs
- Ptosis due to paralysis of the levator.
- Divergence due to unopposed action of the lateral rectus.
- Defective elevation due to paralysis of the superior rectus and inferior oblique muscles (Fig. 259).
- Defective depression due to paralysis of the inferior rectus (Fig. 260).
- Defective adduction due to paralysis of the medial rectus (Fig. 261).
- Intorsion of the eye on attempted downgaze.
- Internal ophthalmoplegia: dilated and unreactive pupil, and defective accommodation.

Fourth nerve palsy

Signs
- Hyperdeviation (latent or manifest) in the primary position.
- Accentuation of hyperdeviation with ipsilateral head tilt (positive Bielschowsky test—Fig. 262).
- Defective depression in adduction (Fig. 263).
- Vertical diplopia worse in downgaze.

Sixth nerve palsy

Signs
- Convergence in the primary position.
- Failure of abduction (Fig. 264).
- Horizontal diplopia worse in abduction.

Causes

- Vascular lesions (hypertension, diabetes): third, fourth, and sixth nerve palsy.
- Posterior communicating aneurysm: painful third nerve palsy with dilated pupil.
- Raised intracranial pressure: bilateral sixth nerve palsy (false localizing sign).
- Trauma: bilateral, fourth nerve palsy and third nerve palsy.
- Cavernous lesions (fistula, thrombosis): fourth and sixth nerve palsy.
- Tumors (acoustic neuroma, nasopharyngeal): sixth nerve palsy.

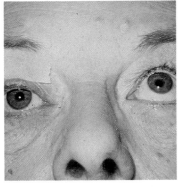

Fig. 259 Right third nerve palsy showing failure of elevation.

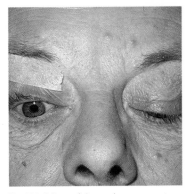

Fig. 260 Failure of depression.

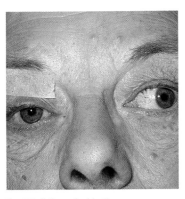

Fig. 261 Failure of adduction.

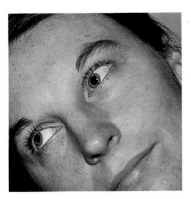

Fig. 262 Positive Bielschowsky test.

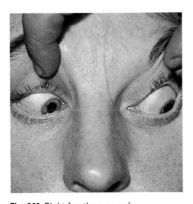

Fig. 263 Right fourth nerve palsy.

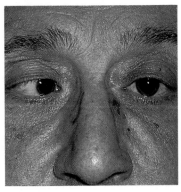

Fig. 264 Left sixth nerve palsy (patient looking to left).

Clinical types

Corneal abrasion

This is usually caused by accidental injuries (e.g., by fingernails, tree branches). It is a painful condition associated with lacrimation and blepharospasm. The epithelial defect, which stains with fluorescein (Fig. 265), usually heals within 24 h. Some patients subsequently develop recurrent corneal erosions.

Treatment: instillation of antibiotic ointment to prevent infection and padding.

Foreign body

- *Subtarsal foreign body.*
- *Corneal ferrous foreign body* may be associated with a rust ring (Fig. 266).
- *Penetrating foreign body* most commonly occurs when metal is being hammered.

Blunt trauma

Apart from blow-out fracture (see Fig. 54), blunt trauma may be associated with the following:

Anterior segment damage
- Subconjunctival hemorrhage and periocular ecchymosis.
- Hyphema (Fig. 267).
- Iris sphincter rupture.
- Iridodialysis (Fig. 268).
- Angle recession (see Fig. 155), which may subsequently lead to chronic glaucoma.
- Lens damage: subluxation (see Fig. 183), dislocation, and cataract formation.
- Scleral rupture is very serious and is usually caused by severe trauma.

Posterior segment damage
- Commotio retinae (Berlin's edema, Fig. 269).
- Choroidal rupture (Fig. 270).
- Retinal tear formation: dialysis, macular hole, or equatorial holes, all of which may result in retinal detachment.

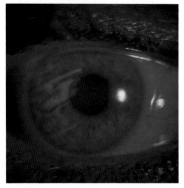

Fig. 265 Corneal abrasion stained with fluorescein.

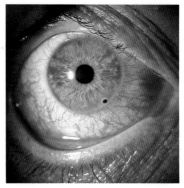

Fig. 266 Corneal foreign body with rust ring.

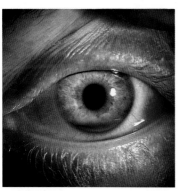

Fig. 267 Hyphema.

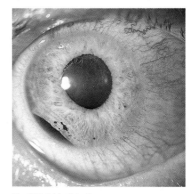

Fig. 268 Iridodialysis.

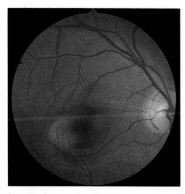

Fig. 269 Commotio retinae.

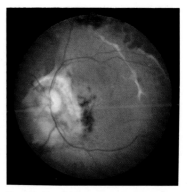

Fig. 270 Choroidal rupture.

Index